To Lynne,

from Myriam Arthur

FORGIVEN

Myriam Arthur

604-850-2747

Produced by:

FriesenPress

Suite 300 – 852 Fort Street
Victoria, BC, Canada V8W 1H8

www.friesenpress.com

Distributed to the trade by The Ingram Book Company

DEDICATIONS

THIS BOOK IS DEDICATED TO THE LOVING MEMORY OF MY SON John Paul.

With many thanks to my husband John for the love and support I always received from him, even more throughout the most vulnerable period in my life.

To our younger son Patrick, my mother and sister, and the rest of my family and friends who never questioned my actions, only supported and loved me.

Lastly I have to thank my friend Chris Rands, who taking time from her busy life proofread my manuscript, correcting some deep-seated errors being that English is my second language.

PROLOGUE

SEPTEMBER 1ST 2009, PASSPORT AND BOARDING TICKING IN HAND I proceeded to the US immigration desk at Canada's Vancouver International Airport. An officer rapidly processed my information, but in a matter of seconds a disdained gaze replaced her previous cordiality. "Someone else will look after you," she said, pointing to a bench for me to sit on.

One hour passed, then two and nothing happened. By now all the passengers of the flight going to Lima via Los Angeles, had gone through immigration. Obviously the flight was on schedule, and I would miss it if someone from Homeland Security didn't get on the ball and allow me through. "What are these people after anyway?" I wondered, my anxiety on the rise.

Finally an officer, who occasionally I'd found glancing at me, called my name. Once I was in front of him in a very mortifying way he said, "You are in violation of the law. You are inadmissible to enter the United States!" His penetrating stare didn't stop as he continued, "Didn't you know that you require the advance permission to enter the United States?"

I was aware of such a requirement, but I had hoped that after these many years our American neighbors would not continue to look through old archives.

"Yes, but the urgency of my trip didn't give me the time. It takes about six months to obtain one; just in case I brought the consent granted to me last year. In addition you should know that my final destination is Lima, Peru where my sister resides. I would just be passing through your country, halting in Los Angeles only to change planes," I responded

Unmoved, the officer said, "Sorry, this permit has expired, you will need to find another route. You'll have to talk to the Arline to make the arrangements." He read a bunch of articles from some papers he retrieved from under the counter and began to ask me all kinds of questions, as if my transgression had happened yesterday instead of more than 20 years ago and more importantly that in happened in another country.

Meanwhile the clock kept ticking and because of the fashion in which my ticket was issued, I could easily lose the chance to make the appropriate changes in my itinerary.

"Do you do understand all I have read to you and my questions?" he barked, handing me a pen and pointing repeatedly to the place where my name was printed. "If so, sign now here. Once this is completed, I will call the Royal Canadian Mountain Police to escort you off our premises.

Of course I understood all his rhetoric and I had no choice but to sign, though I found it absurd, uncompassionate, as well as humiliating. Some minutes later two RCMP marched by my side doing their duty, they removed an undesirable traveler from the United States compound, back to the departure area, just a few meters away.

COCHABAMBA-BOLIVIA, JUNE 1985

NOT A CLOUD IN THE SKY, EVEN WITH WINTER SETTLING IN, NOT at all unusual in Cochabamba, my native city. Other than today the sun seemed brighter and warmer, extra special because our "number one son," as I sometimes cheerily called him, was arriving from California.

John Paul, not quite 24, had completed his studies. He now held a Bachelor Degree in Fine Arts from the University of Southern California. J.P. had kept us informed on his progress, also about the fantastic job he got as a Makeup Artist with Universal Studios. It was a post that ignited a new dream in him; he now planned to broaden his studies in Special Effects to become a Director, following in the footsteps of Steven Spielberg.

We could not complain; our investments of the past few years had paid off. They not only enabled us to send our son to the States and pay for his studies in a well known university in California, but to also have John Paul come home on his breaks. Yet it did not matter how often we had him back, in each and every one of his visits he brought an invigorating joy. There was an even greater reason to rejoice and celebrate now; he had just graduated! So here we were at the airport, my husband John and I, our younger son Patrick and several of JP's friends impatiently waiting for his arrival.

1

The minute I saw J.P. I was elated with pride. The California suntan and the well-trimmed beard framing his face enhanced his looks; self-assurance radiated throughout all his pores. Approaching closer to us, JP's pace changed to a run, and within seconds I was lifted up in his arms and tenderly hugged and kissed. He then went to his brother and gave him a bear hug, not brutal enough to hurt him, but powerfully strong. Patrick took it without a blink. John was treated with a bit more respect; he received a manly embrace together with a kiss on his cheek.

The Hollywood setting where John Paul lately spent much of his time, didn't appear to have changed our son. At an age where life was a continuous adventure, J.P. not only cared a lot for the entire family, but also was not embarrassed to openly show his affection. Everything in John Paul was passionate, his laughter, his love, even his sadness. John Paul's outgoing personality captivated everyone. He was a hero to Patrick, who at fourteen, loved him to pieces, affection entirely reciprocated by his brother.

Very popular with the opposite sex was even considered an eligible catch, but as far as I knew JP. had no one special in his life. If the subject ever came up, our son jokingly said, "I'm waiting for someone special Mom; someone like you!" and would dismiss the topic, laughing and hugging me.

Now our son was home, but between work, parties, friends coming and going, we hardly had a quiet moment in our household; my husband's and my own latest pursuits did not leave much opportunity for intimate family moments. One day, taking advantage of a break, John Paul with a stern look on his face told me, "Will you slow down Mom? I need to talk with you, in private!"

His request didn't surprise or worry me. John Paul and I had always had a wonderful mother and son relationship. Frequently we had friendly discussions during which he would confide his thoughts and dreams. Laid-back now, I thought he was going to tell me he found the girl of his dreams, or perhaps something related to his studies. Therefore, carefree, I sat down to chat.

Then I heard my son hoarsely say, "Mom, I suspect I have been infected with AIDS. Don't ask me any questions Mom, just help me please!" A silent roar behind my son's cry for help followed.

Stunned as if hit by lightning, I kept quiet. In a haze I thought, *This can't be! I must have heard wrong.* Except that when I looked at John Paul to ask him to repeat what he had just said, there was no need, my son's pale and troubled face confirmed it all.

Unable to utter a word, my mind, my ears, my whole being kept hearing the statement repeating itself over and over, "I'm infected with AIDS, I'm infected with AIDS." Surely it had to be a nightmare, but it was not; it was real. I kept mute.

What could I have said anyway? The little I knew about AIDS was what I had read in some sensational magazines stating that the virus was fatal, information that pierced my mind now. Those lurid publications even printed malicious gossip surrounding the recently discovered disease, stating that it was mainly transmitted among homosexuals.

No one knew much about it; the outbreak was still too fresh. No qualified source or any media attempted to express a serious opinion on the topic. Homosexual lifestyles were blamed, followed by a hateful public backlash against gays.

Surely my son needed some reassurance from me, but instead those articles stating that AIDS was a deadly disease kept banging on my brain. The thought that I could lose John Paul was unbearable; my two sons were the reason for my existence. To know AIDS was fatal was agony enough, but to think it mainly struck the homosexual population compounded the woe.

Why? I was not sure. In my city full of *macho* men, only disgust was shown to who ever gave signs of being homosexual and I was afraid for my son, and for our family.

Tortured by these thoughts, I tightly held my son's hands, desperately trying to fight back my tears and speak. I had to tell him how much I loved him no matter what, but no words came from my mouth.

The rush of my blood going through my brain seemed thunderous, yet only a profound silence surrounded us; for how long, seconds or minutes, I don't know. Worse yet, John Paul's helplessness was still out in the open and I could not do or say anything.

I sensed he was not looking only for help. I believe what he wanted more than anything was to share his sorrow with someone who would understand the enormity of his pain. But before I could say a word, he regained control and in a commanding voice told me, "Mom, you have to promise not to tell a word of this to my father. I can't bear the thought! Oh, please Mom, just don't tell him anything; at least until I'm certain I have the disease!" I had the feeling he spoke those last words just in an attempt to ease the concern he saw in my face.

Coming out of my daze, I finally heard myself speak. But considering the depth of our tragedy my words of assurance and love I directed to my son sounded meaningless.

After John Paul confided in me, I feigned a migraine headache and remained locked in my room. I was hoping for a cataclysm to strike so that I would not have to face the next day, let alone the future, but all I got were more questions.

I vaguely remembered reading about Rock Hudson's story. In the early part of 1985, when it was made public that he had AIDS; rumor has it that for some time but it was a well-kept secret. A few other articles referred to the numerous trips he made to France in search of a cure and later reporters even wrote about his homosexual lifestyle.

Was my son homosexual? Was this the reason he got infected? John Paul had never given any indication, and I didn't have the courage to inquire any deeper, "Don't ask me anything Mom," he had said! Cowardly I accepted and respected his plea. Besides what relevance did these questions have anyway? That my son's life was in peril was the only thing that mattered.

But then again, I knew that if anyone learned John Paul was infected, it would lead people to think, "If he has contracted that horrifying disease, it has to be because he is homosexual." In a society dominated by male chauvinism where men brought about their *machismo* through muscles and fights or by who broke more girls' hearts, there would be finger-pointing or worse.

John Paul was well built, had a muscular body but he was also refined, he hated fights and was artistically inclined. My son loved the opposite sex but also respected them; we just had to be careful about the whole thing, gossip was cruel.

The thought that it could become voice *populi* terrified me, also angered me. I had seen a friend's family emotionally destroyed by gossip and slander. It happened after the Hudson lifestyle story was out in the open. Encouraged by the acknowledgment, our friend's brother decided to publicly declare he was a homosexual, the despise and rejection was brutal.

In my hometown you just don't say things like that without causing a scandal. I could not let that ever happen to us. It would be devastating. I not only had to protect John Paul but also the rest of my family. The secret had to remain between my son and I; not even his father could know. It was what John Paul had asked of me in the first place.

Not because his father was a *machista*, like most of Bolivian men were. No! J. P. knew his Dad was the kindest and gentlest person in the world, even if he played with guns and loved to hunt. He also knew John loved him and would not hesitate to kill anyone who dared tried to hurt either one of his sons, after all he was from Western Canada, the land of cowboys.

John Paul's request likely came because he felt self-conscious, and I kept silent because my son didn't need to be mortified any further. Besides, I also felt guilty. It was me who had sprung the idea to send our son to study in California and made it happened, perhaps when John Paul was too young to fend for himself. Above and beyond I had in mind to fix the problem first , as if it could be fixable!

All were petty matters in excruciating circumstances, unworthy of my Christian up-bringing, but then again, focused on the success of our businesses, engaged in corporate parties in entertaining a lot I'd already wandered off, far from God.

As a result, now perplexed with my pain, I went so far as to blame Him for our son's misfortune. "Why are you doing this to us? If I have angered you, why didn't you direct your anger towards me, not by afflicting my son?" I dared to ask this unmerciful God.

The thought I could lose John Paul frightened me. So I continued to address Him with a raging spirit: "You have no right to do this to us!" I was letting fear, a low-down advisor, take control of my mind.

Thankfully John was away in the field; had he been home I don't know what I would have said to him to explain my sobbing of the night. At one point I must have dozed off and I was still wrapped up in the warmth of my migraine flight, when the first rays of dawn trickling in through the blinds brought back the crushing pain of my son's news. More alert now, I realized that being sorry for myself didn't solve anything and from the Hudson story, I concluded that John Paul required immediate medical attention.

Yet with some gaps in the information that still needed to be filled, a couple of days later when J. P. and I were alone again, I asked him, "Why are you certain you have AIDS, John Paul?" When my son first had confided in me he had not revealed much. Now I hoped he would tell me more.

J.P. didn't respond immediately, but after a moment of silence, likely realizing I had the right to know somberly said, "I am not sure what exactly happened Mom. As far as I know while in Los Angeles, I engaged in unprotected sex with prostitutes. They must have carried the virus, because a few months later, I began to have peculiar symptoms: fever, swelling of some of my lymph nodes, specially under my arm pits and neck, some nausea and vomiting. I was told that this were the apparent consequences of being infected."

"Did you have any tests done to confirm your suspicion son?" For a while seemed that John Paul did not want to say anything anymore, but seconds later in a whisper he added, "Yes; but I was lonely and scared. I hardly knew anything about AIDS, except that it was deadly and if I tested positive, I would not have been able to cope with such a diagnosis on my own. I didn't wait for the results. I decided to come home instead."

I could see how difficult it was for my son to reflect on his ordeal. Again I backed away and did not pursue any further with my interrogation. I just embraced my son, while my heart ached for him.

It appeared that J.P. and I were equally ignorant on the subject of HIV/AIDS. It was early on the 80s, and the research was still in infancy; the amount of accurate information we had about the diseases' causes and effects was minimal. Had I had access to the information the World Health Organization or the many other associations now provide about the disease, I would have realized that John Paul had contracted HIV, which later could develop to AIDS; the knowledge would have enlightened me, preventing the irrationality of some of my actions, the many mistakes I made and the pain and anxiety I caused. Unfortunately at the time no such resources were available.

Silently I went over my son's words; "I engaged in unprotected sex with prostitutes, I must have contracted it from them." In my view those prostitutes necessarily had to be females, and for some reason the statement lifted some of the weight I carried; my son was not homosexual.

Not that I ever had anything against gay people. No, I actually held in high esteem the few I knew, but I was still relieved. I suppose my father's rigid upbringing on the topic must have rubbed into my inner core; he was a man who thought very little of homosexuals and perhaps this could have narrowed my outlook

I had no other conversations of this sort with my son. I just began to explore a fast way to have him cured. But where? Our situation was complex; we were well known in my city, but it was imperative I promptly obtain guidance on what steps to take. Perhaps I could entrust George with our secret, and if anyone, he would be the one to direct my search. He was a distant relative and a physician. I shared my thoughts with John Paul. He reluctantly accepted the idea.

I first went to see George alone and after I explained all I knew about my son's condition, I asked him, "Will you help me, George? I don't know what to do, or where to go. Please give me an idea?" Caught off guard with my problem, it took George a few minutes to respond. "Bring your son tomorrow. I'll open up early. I want to check him and run some tests on him before I recommend anything," he finally said with a sympathetic tone in his voice

The next day John Paul went by himself. At his return he reported, "Dr. Moreno examined me, but didn't say much. He ordered different blood tests, which were done in the lab next door. I'm supposed to return next week; he will have the results back by then. At that point, I want you to come with me. Personally, I don't think he can do much for me, nor give us any other news than what I have already told you. It's best you are there to hear what Dr. Moreno has to say."

"Of course I will go, John Paul," I said convinced George was going to perform wonders. I was even confident that the blood work would negate that my son had been infected.

Time marched unnervingly slow, but on the day of the appointment full of the same conviction I went with J.P. The minute we got in, George uneasily said, "John Paul's tests are back, some of the symptoms as well as the results from the blood work make me suspect an infection has occurred, but that is all. Unfortunately here in Bolivia we lack specialized technology to positively identify the virus; we haven't even begun to scratch the surface in this field." George's tenseness mounted as he continued, "I'm terribly sorry, Myriam, but it is impossible for me to give J.P. a diagnosis."

My face plastered with disappointment must have moved George, because with genuine concern he added, "I believe France is right now the most advanced country in the research, closely followed by the United States. A treatment, if not the cure, must be available by now in either country. John Paul should be examined and tested over there." Unable to do anything more for us, emphatically he wished us good luck. J.P. and I thanked him for his advice and left.

It could not have been a bigger letdown for me. I had hoped for so much. On our way home, John Paul kept quiet. He didn't say, "I told you so, Mom." We were both just sad. But George had also presented a solution; it was now up to me to take action. I suspected my son was not too eager to return to the States, Since George had also highlighted France, I began to consider that possibility.

An important element for the equation was money; a trip abroad, as vital as it was, came with a very high price tag. John's own cancer experience from a few years back had taught us the magnitude of medical costs out of the country and currently we didn't have that kind of liquidity.

The decree to re-establish democracy in Bolivia had created political chaos and a rampant inflation gripped our nation's economy, which together with the international crisis ended by bankrupting Bolivia. As a result our own finances were not in great shape either; it would be a delusion to try and secure any money in the present state of affairs.

The regime that for the past 10 years had ruled the country, as strange as it may seem, had provided a sense of security. The official exchange of $ 20 Bolivian pesos for 1 US dollar had not fluctuated, but now the political unrest created an imbalance.

An unreasonable demand for the American currency flooded the banks. It was a normal reaction from people in panic, but a vicious circle began the more the demand increased, the more the exchange rate escalated. All transactions as well as bank loans operated only in American dollars; several companies were forced to close operations.

The chaos caused moral values to change, corporations, companies and persons in general traded in the black market exchange. It didn't make any difference that this market derived from drug money; the general consensus was that drug traffickers supported what was left of the Bolivian economy. Life and business had to go on; working people had to be paid.

Of course the mayhem had impacted our two industries as well. Contracts at the factory had diminished; luxury items such as marble items and floors were not a necessity. Even our construction venture went into hibernation. Uncertainty surrounded us, yet for some unknown reason we didn't take the problem seriously and John and I continued to entertain and drink a lot.

By 1985 the rate of exchange skyrocketed to 2.5 million *pesos Bolivianos* for one American dollar. With this ballooning inflation, money in my country became worthless, comparable only to the inflation which occurred in Germany after W.W.II.

Under these circumstances is when John Paul came home.

corner of the room away from my friends, to keep the promise I made to myself to be well behaved.

The nuns had a weekly procedure to make parents aware of their offspring's demeanor; each Monday we received report cards on the past week's behavior. For excellent conduct, white ones were handed out, blue for good, green for a questionable behavior and yellow meant immediate dismissal from school for a three days period. The cards were to be returned by the next day, signed by our parents! My consistencies were the blues.

May was a significant month; the 27th was Mother's day. It was important I obtained a white card every week, for the entire month. I had in mind to give them to my Mom as a present and I was not going to let Madre Hortencia spoil my gift. It was vital I keep silent.

How did I dream up this anyway? I knew it would be difficult, with the playful and talkative reputation my sister and I had in school. "Remember this is the reason Myriam; you have to prove you can do it," I told myself. Somehow I had to vindicate our history; my sister Vicky, from very small was very active, con-tinuously on the go and was a motive of panic for the nuns and I had not been a saint either. But today, Madre Hortencia was just plain unjust!

Be honest Myriam, I reminded myself. You gave the nuns more than enough reasons to make them suspect you were the insti-gator of the mischief. Remember the time when you and Sylvia were hiding in the storage room, behind the old piano because you didn't want to attend mass? Of course I remembered. But why did they have to force us to go to mass every morning in the first place and make us kneel down on the hard ceramic tiles for most of the whole observance. That was not a celebration it was more like a martyrdom preparation; we purposely hid behind the old piano and manipulated the piano keys, as if a ghost played it, to scare Madre Leticia. Frightened she immediately got other nuns involved in the phantom search and found us, instead!

How about the time when we both caught a few wasps, removed their stingers and replaced them with tiny love notes to *Cupido*. Then the whole swarm, the ones with the notes and the ones without, got furious and in revenge began to attack everyone in the chemistry room. Madre Elvira was not too happy about it, and you and Silvia had to face the music. You should be thankful you didn't get ousted from school. Yes, of course I know I am not a saint, but it does not give *madre* Hortencia the right to be so *injusta*. This time I was not doing anything, just swimming against the current, trying to prove a point.

"Myriam be quiet." Madre Hortencia said interrupting my thoughts, and not even looking back to see whom was doing the talking. I felt the sting in my tongue as I gnawed it to keep silent. With my head down, I just continued doing the task she had demanded from us, but next to me the buzzing noise increased. Girls from another group were horsing around taking advantage of the fact the nun had her back towards us, writing some notes on the blackboard.

She abruptly turned around and with a commanding voice told me, "Myriam this is the last warning I'm giving to you. You either keep quiet or you are out of my class." This time I could not accept the injustice so I answered back "But mother Hortencia, it's not me who is talking. Why don't you open your eyes and check before you accuse me of something I'm not doing?"

"I have had enough with you Myriam; you are even talking back to me now. You best get out of my class right now. I'll report you later to the *Prefecta*." And she pointed to the door.

At that moment I truly lost it! I forgot my good intentions. Angered I stood up and stomped out of the room, and once out, I furiously slammed the door, almost in *Madre Hortencia's* face. Bad, more than just bad, this was really bad; it had been a horrendous mistake. The second hour I was called to the *Prefecta's* office and not allowing me to explain anything, I was suspended from school for the entire week.

to connect with the opposite sex without being too obvious. Suddenly out of nowhere, the same young man we left at the store was in front of us introducing himself, "My name is John Arthur, and I come from Canada; what is yours?" he asked, smiling.

I supposed his friendly physiognomy and wide smile forced me to answer. "Mine is Myriam and this is my friend Fernanda." Encouraged by my response, he went a little further. He actually muttered an invitation! "Shall we go for a drive? Would you please join me? We could go for a drink or an ice cream; just say yes! Please?" He acted as if he were a dear old friend, requesting our company.

Of course it was out of the question, so I said, "No thank you. Good-bye." He didn't budge. Just then Fernanda made me notice the noise around us. The honking and commotion came from the line of cars detained behind a taxi; it was the cab John had jumped out of to talk to us. Naturally the driver was not about to move it until the crazy customer was back in.

The street was congested for more than a block, everyone honking impatiently. My friend and I were embarrassed. We had not chosen to be the center of this comical scene. "What to do? We could say yes to this persistent foreigner or no and continue to be the cause of the unwanted turmoil. Fernanda and I looked at each other and laughing accepted, got in the taxi and went for an ice cream.

Once at the ice cream parlor, this Canadian young man continued to talk, "I've come to Bolivia to do exploratory work in the jungles of your country Myriam. I work for an American Geophysical firm in search of oil fields." John spoke mainly in English, but slow and with the odd word in Spanish, which made easy for me to understand. He was young and good looking; he seemed intelligent and except for being 5'6"instead of 6' he was almost perfect.

My thoughts were interrupted by his next words, "I've seen you several times before, but I was never able to approach you. Today, I wasn't going to lose sight of you again," he explained and insisted, "I had been in love with you from the first time I saw you." I took all this as a joke, however we did became good friends. John, a Geological Engineer, was enjoying his second day of leave from camp.

From then on, this fervent admirer always made sure I knew the next time he would be in town. "I work twenty-one days in the field and I have ten days off in the city. I'll come to visit you the minute I'm out," John said smiling, not in the least expecting a "No." From then on, when in town he regularly came to our house.

He was well liked by my parents, especially by my father. Sometimes I would come home from my courses, only to find him happily visiting my father, forgetting he had come to see me. John's persistence and affability won us all over, even my mother, who at first reluctantly accepted him. It must have been the flowers he never failed to bring her that prompted the success!

Then December arrived and I found only natural to invite John over for Christmas Eve, a time for anyone away from home likely to be homesick. We celebrated Christmas in a traditional family fashion, first we attended the midnight Mass, followed by a late supper; presents were opened right after. All keyed up, John accepted.

The church was only a block a way from our house. After the service, a full moon crowned the night, and thousands of sparkling stars hung over the firmament as we walked back home. John taking me aside from my parents, lovingly and showing me a beautiful ring in a question form said, "Myriam, please marry me?" Caught by surprise, I didn't know what to say. We had known each other for no more than two months; I had not even thought we were dating.

What I didn't know is that because John came from another culture, between scenes he thought he had to win my father over, so he asked first his permission, "I'm in love with you daughter Don Guillermo. I would like to marry her." My father responded, "John, have you asked her? I have nothing to do with it; it must be solely her decision."

The stillness of the night, the stars and the moon probably had a lot to do with what I was about to say, but mainly because the *gringuito* I had decreed I would marry in my early teens was actually asking me to be his wife, and all I had to do to make it happen was to say "Yes!"

So I did.

Soon after his work took him back to the jungle. For a newly engaged bride to be, John's time away, was like living in an imaginary dream. Besides it only now dawned on me that I hardly knew this man I was to marry on May 5th. But the big date was still five months ahead; a lot of things could happen until then, and they did.

The exploration in Bolivia ended ahead of time. The entire crew was to return to the headquarters in the U.S.A. before the original date. Chaos ensued and our plans had to change. John wanted to marry me immediately, whereas I tried to buy more time nervously saying half English, half Spanish, "*Amor,* why don't you go ahead and when you know where your company will send you, you come back *por mi.*"

John understood it all, the cold feet included, and didn't accept my suggestion. Nor was he about to compromise either. Instead John firmly said, "You marry me now, or never!" I got the picture too and my heart chose to say, "Okay, I will." Yet I didn't like what was happening, to proceed with the new plan everything had to be changed, starting with the wedding date. It had to be moved ahead. The only one available in our parish was February 17th and the date could not have been more inopportune.

It happened to be in the mist of my fertile time and as a Catholic the only method to prevent conception was to avoid having sexual intercourse during that period. At this particular time and age it would have been more than improper to discuss such a subject with your fiancé, and in our honeymoon, I could not just tell my future hubby, "Honey, lets not have sex now, just pretend we did, Okay!"

Ha, ha. Even in my present quandary, I could not stop laughing thinking of the face John would put on at such a request! There was nothing I could do about it, so I just continued forward telling myself, "If is the will of God, let it happen."

My sister and Raul barely made it home before the wedding day arrived. Hit by the reality I would soon be leaving all that was dear to me, around 5pm I considered playing the role of the runaway bride and disappear. By 7pm, encouraged by my sister, I came to my senses and made it to the church on time.

The décor was superb: pink magnolias and roses throughout the altar and small bouquets on the bench side of the main passageway. My parents and sister had put great love into the decorating and the result was irresistible. Lead by my father I glided down the aisle dressed in a beautiful white gown; Verdi's nuptial march skillfully played masked the sound of my heart's beat. John more handsome than ever dressed in his tuxedo, waited for me by the altar. Mass was celebrated and once it ended, John and I spoke our vows.

After the service my parents held a banquet at their home. Only close friends and relatives were the guests, but the number exceeded a hundred. The gathering was not only to celebrate our wedding, but also to bid us farewell. The next day we were leaving the country; one of the reasons for my panic.

Certainly I was excited, but also frightened; tomorrow was the start of my new life as Mrs. Myriam Arthur. My husband and I were going away to create a home of our own; no idea where this might be yet. If John was not satisfied with what his company had to offer, it would be Canada, This meant cold and snowy winters; interesting but also intimidating spoiled as I was by the mild climate in my hometown.

The language was my other big concern; my English still needed a good workout! John, aware of my apprehensions assured me, "Darling I love you so much. You don't need to worry about anything. You'll see the great life we'll have together, wherever this might happen to be."

Early in the morning thunder and lightning woke us up, which was normal at this time of the year; it was the rainy season. The overcast continued throughout the day and our flight from Cochabamba to La Paz's international airport booked for 11 am was first postponed and later canceled. Luckily our journey to Miami from La Paz was booked for the 19ᵗʰ in the afternoon, which was the next day.

After another glorious day and night in Cochabamba, the next morning the sky was clear and our flight took off. In La Paz, as I presented my passport to board the plane to Florida, I had an unexpected obstacle; emigration officers stopped me saying, "*Lo siento señora, usted no puede salir del país.*" No further explanation. John and I almost had heart attacks. The agents adamantly were opposed to letting me leave the country.

Recuperated from the initial shock, John and I simultaneously asked, "Why *Porqué, que pasa?*" The officer in command coldly responded, "*La fecha de salida estampada en su pasaporte esta equivocada,*" True, the date stamped in my document read February 18ᵗʰ, and it was now the 19ᵗʰ. We had overlooked this minor detail that now generated a major problem. The rule imposed by the political party in power was that every Bolivian citizen leaving the country had to have the departure date stamped in the passport; it worked as *salvo conducto* for political control.

It was impossible to have that stupid date renewed. It would take more than two hours just to get to the governmental offices in La Paz's centre, not counting the time for the drive back; we would miss our flight. We tried to convince the officers to ignore the slip-up and let me go, but they maintained their negative mode.

We were almost ready to give up, when a friend passing by saw our predicament. High in rank in the political arena Renato asked, "What seems to be the problem John?" My husband made him immediately aware of the situation and Renato suggested, "You only need to pay the guys a few pesos and they will let Myriam board the plane." John had thought of that himself, except that afraid to offend the officers and create more delays he'd closed that avenue. Now following our friend's advice, my husband handed them over all the Bolivian money he had in his pockets: no more than one hundred dollars. It solved our crisis.

Once in Calgary, John often liked to blow his own horn and used this piece of my history as conversational material. "You have no idea what I had to do to get my wife off the hook from Bolivian authorities. Emigration officials wouldn't let Myriam leave her country, so I had to bribe them. I paid a lot of money for her!" And he'd chuckle as he finished telling the tale.

It irritated me a bit, so I in turn using an anecdote he revealed about his mom, I like to tease him too. When John and I started to date he had mentioned his parents knew very little about Bolivia and its people. Realizing her son would be working in that area, Margaret, John's mom dug an old Encyclopedia Britannica and gathered some facts. She found that three major groups of natives lived in Bolivia: the *Aimaras* who had their settlements in higher elevations, the *Guaranies* in the low lands, and the *Quechuas* who built the Inca Empire; their domain was in the valleys; my area.

The encyclopedia portrayed the natives dressed in their traditional clothes, as hundreds of years ago. Males wore colorful garland feathers on their heads, nothing on their torsos, and something like a short skirt covered their sex part; females wore also the feathers plus bright colorful skirts. Nothing was mentioned in the book about the whites, the descendants of the Spanish *conquistadores,* who were also part of the Bolivian heritage, and apparently John didn't bother to correct the omission.

Then came the day when John told his parents he was engaged to a Bolivian girl; his Mom had probably wondered, "Is my son's fiancé one of those native people?" The words in the letter she wrote to him reflected it. "Son, if **that** is what you want, we shall be happy for you. You have our blessings," Which echoed to me that she so loved her son that his choosing would not affect her love. I was to meet John's parents soon; it made me nervous.

Nervousness was a mode I didn't like to linger in, so I decided to have some fun hiding my anxiety in the anecdote, "Honey, your mama must be a special lady; she accepted me even with feathers and all. Should I wear my garland when we get there? I brought it; I have it in my suitcase," I joked and laughed, while silently I prayed to be truly accepted by his parents.

In a whirlpool of excitement for the past twenty days, I had not finished adjusting to one place yet and there we were, jumping into another. I still had in my pores the warmth from the ten incredible days of leisure time I had with my husband in Daytona Beach, where we spent part of our honeymoon, sunbathing and having some dips in the waters of the Atlantic Ocean. Winter was well entrenched in the northern hemisphere, but not yet in Florida.

Nor in our next stop Jackson, Mississippi, John's company's headquarters. Soaring heat and humidity, similar to the tropics in my country, hit us here; only continuous cold showers and ice cold drinks helped me battle the heat. Our stay was short. My husband had no interest in what the company had to offer him, so we continued to Calgary, via Chicago and Edmonton.

In Chicago as we descended from the plane the weather changed, it was snowing. Since all I knew about Chicago came from the big screen. movies about gangsters, Italians, and night-clubs, industries, and smog I decided to have a dive into that worldly life. We had a couple of days' wait in what to me seemed a most intriguing city. So giving into an outright curiosity, I asked John, "Honey, I've never been in a striptease club, will you take me to one, please?" My husband, who had not yet stopped pleas-ing me, accepted my request.

My inquisitiveness didn't pay off. Not one hour later I changed my appeal, "Let's leave! I don't want to stay here a minute longer. How dare that half naked woman provocatively approach you? She even sat on your lap and you let her. Why didn't you send her away? Instead you just smiled; you probably even enjoyed it," I said, furiously jealous. Surprised by my sudden outburst, my husband had no choice but pay for the drinks, collect our coats, and leave the place.

Our stay in Chicago was short. Not because of my tantrum, no. It was because we had an itinerary to follow. The next day we flew to Edmonton, my official landing entry into Canada; or, in my view, the entrance to the North Pole. Brrr... Brrr...my teeth rattled as I stepped out of the plane. It was March, everything was covered with snow and the sub-zero temperature took my breath away. I never expected to be entering a deepfreeze, but here I was!

midday meal, it was 11 am. While no more than 20 feet away, water flowing into cement sinks from fixed faucets on the wall, men with naked torsos tended to their personal hygiene. Further back other prisoners appear to be exercising, while others yet, walked in between barrels of garbage, from where the unpleasant smell reaching our nostrils seemed to emanate.

Protected by the iron bars, apprehensive and sickened by the sight, my husband and I observed. It was more like something out of one of Dante's scenarios. Overwhelmed I suggested, "John lets go. We have no business being here." Too late, the two Americans were now at the other side.

A sentinel came out from a cubbyhole and unlocked the gate to let us in, locking it right back behind us. We were now out in the open with the rest of the inmate population. John protectively held my hand, while not the least intimidated reached the other out to greet the Americans, "Hello young fellows; I'm John Arthur," my husband said, with a sincere smile on his face. His greeting gave me courage and I followed his example saying, "I'm his wife, Myriam."

Addressing them in English helped break barriers. I saw relief and hope spread in their faces. "I'm Jim Bennett and this is my friend Darryl Martin, one of them said smiling. "We have been in this place for the past four months for possession of cocaine. We are supposed to be tried, but we don't know when." Jim looked about twenty, or twenty one, Darryl a little older.

Jim then asked us, "Do you mind coming upstairs? We could have more privacy to talk there. Besides, it would be interesting to find out what you guys think of our quarters" No guards made any attempt to stop us. We gathered there was no protocol to follow and climbed a flight of stairs; it took us to the upper balcony.

Escorted by the two Americans and supported by John's arm, I walked through uneven inlaid brick floors seemingly worn out by time, into one of the hallways that trailed into the building. It ended in to what appeared to be a large room, but pieces of wood, bricks and cardboard divided the area into small cubicles, giving inmates a reduce amount of privacy. The boys had no beds, only two old mattresses tossed on the floor and a couple of small wooden boxes that served as tables or sitting places. Apparently most living areas shared similar characteristics.

Shocked, I gasped. John with a concern look on his face asked, "Is here where you sleep then?" "Yes, but the worst part is that we don't have any money to purchase the bare necessities. In the States we saved a whole year's wages to come to Bolivia. We heard that weed, cocaine, and other stuff were dirt cheap; we wanted to experiment. We experimented all right and spent all our money! We were having a great time until the law caught up with us. We have an appointed public lawyer for our defense, but he hasn't done much; as you can see we are still here."

Touched by what Jim said, their surroundings, and their age I inquired, "Would you give us the lawyer's name, maybe we can help you on that. People sometimes need a little push to get things done." Jim wrote the name and handed the paper over to my husband.

Now John asked again, "Jim is anything else you need? Are there restrictions as to what we could bring to help out?"

"Oh yah, we would love to have some toilet paper. It's a luxury here. We have been wiping with newspaper papers; sorry about the disgusting subject, but it's the truth. Some cigarettes would also be great, we don't smoke, but we can exchange them for something else. No, there are no restrictions, but it's not a good idea to bring too much at one time; the other tenants might tend to claim it as theirs." Both boys chuckled after Jim's words. I suppose they'd learned to look at their situation with humor.

John and I visited Jim and Darryl every other week, bringing them the requested items, plus bread and some canned goods. John spoke to their lawyer, even paid him a few dollars so that he was more diligent in looking after their case. Three months later the boys were set free. Darryl went home to the States. Jim stayed in Cochabamba. He had been dating a girl from my hometown and married her when he got out. Occasionally they visited us, but it had been at least a couple of years since I last saw Jim.

While his imprisonment we visited Jim simply out of the goodness of our hearts, but I was now seeking his whereabouts with ulterior motives.

MARCH, 1960

INSIDE THE CAB, I TOLD MY HUSBAND SHIVERING, "I'M FREEZING! I feel like a penguin without its tuxedo coat. You never told me it was this cold?" My wardrobe, of course unsuited for a winter in Canada, certainly didn't help matters. Understanding my irritation John said the magic words "Don't worry honey, I'll take you shopping soon." Hugging me he sealed his promise with a kiss.

With the drive to his place, the more I believed I had arrived at the North Pole; literally everything was covered with snow and the fluffy cotton flakes kept coming down! Back home, that white stuff was seen only at the peak of the mountains. Our winters were exceptionally mild, usually characterized by blue skies and a radiant sun, which spoiled all people from Cochabamba. Tobogganing or to play in the snow was an added feature, but one had to drive miles, then hike up some hundred meters or more to achieve the goal. Once the excitement was worn-out, the snow was left behind and we returned to the warmth of the city. Not here, the entire outdoors seemed like a deepfreeze!

Weather shocked, I fiercely held my husband's arm while I shut my eyes with fright! I had to do it. The taxi driver seemed a maniac as he drove through the slippery roads, missing oncoming vehicles by a hairline. I must confess however, the drive went smoothly. The thrilling experience lasted for over one hour, the time it took to get to my husband's place. Thankfully we didn't hit anyone, nor did any of the other cars hit us. The experience forced me to think, "Canadians must be born with special sensory organs that gives them the driving expertise!" I didn't see any other explanation for such precise maneuvering

John's Mom, who knew we were coming, probably heard the car and no sooner were we out from the cab, my husband was in his mother's arms; hugged and kissed over and over. As we entered the house Margaret politely tried to give me the time of the day too, but her attention was mainly on her son. "Oh darling, I've missed you so much. You'd never imagine how much."

She then began to cry. My husband was the younger of her two sons. She had lost her first husband, father of Kenneth and John, when my husband was only two. Ten years later Margaret married Gordon, who helped her raise the boys. They had no other children.

A bit calmer now, Margaret still talking to John said, "You are back now and that's all that matters, I'm so happy; I think I'll cry again." My husband seizing her by the shoulders and laughing said, "No Mom, please don't!"

I was also prone to tears, besides that already I had started to fill home sick and before I knew it, I began to sob. Collecting some courage, trying to joke a little and break the moment, in my broken English I said, "Would your tears be from relief Margaret?" My mother in-law frowning quizzically looked at me in an attempt to process my statement. Pointing to my forehead I clarified, "I'm not wearing the feathers you expected to see on my head!" More puzzled yet, she raised her eyebrows.

John, who knew what I was trying to say, immediately put a light on the subject and explained to his Mom the anecdote of the old encyclopedia and Margaret began to laugh. I believe the tears and the laugher brought our hearts closer. While all our emotions were still afloat, Gordon arrived. John introduced us and he soon joined in the joviality. It was the start of a wonderful relationship. I had been accepted!

A few days later my prince charming and I went on a hunt in search for a place to live and we found a cozy, furnished one-bedroom apartment close to all amenities. It quickly became clear that I was to manage it.

Did he actually expect me to do it? Silently I had to laugh. It wasn't that I was a brat. No! But before, it was my mother together with our maid that took care of those chores. I had no idea about planning or cooking meals, nor laundering, let alone cleaning.

Therefore every day was a challenge. I was often excited, baffled, or both. John never complained, His tolerance reassured me that my deficits were not that important. Somehow after burning a few meals, I managed to present something decent for my husband to eat.

In the blink of an eye many changes kept happening in my life; now this loving *gringuito*, who was my husband, my playmate, and the sole decision maker in our household, found a job. He was contracted as a Drilling Fluids and Trouble-shooter Engineer, a long title that apparently fitted well with his expertise, but that took him away from me.

In charge of some oil fields through Alberta and northern British Columbia, John drove hundreds of kilometers per day. If a drilling problem arose, he was forced to stay at a well site for a day or two and even more. The situation was not too comforting for me, since I was left home alone.

Canada was still a foreign country to me and without John I felt totally at loss. Besides, my English was not as good as I thought it was. Studying it was one thing, but listening and speaking it 24/7 was utterly a nightmare. I ended with horrible headaches and this barrier kept me to some extent isolated. Consequently I clung tightly to the person I loved, my husband, even if it might have seemed somewhat childish.

More so since I had prided myself in having an adventurous spirit. Seeing far away places and meet new people had been always in my dreams, but seemingly I had not finished growing up. All was great if John was by my side, but it was a different story when he was gone and for far longer than expected. At that point I would panic. I imagined him in a car accident, badly hurt, bleeding, and no one would come to his rescue; cellular phones were not even a flash in an inventor's imagination just yet.

What's more, I was in my second month of pregnancy, the result of the unexpected wedding date change. John was unaware yet, and I still didn't show signs. So afraid for my husband, but also because of my own insecurity, I insistently asked him, "Honey, please take me with you. I'm terrified when you are not here with me. You can do it; after all you are your own boss."

"Myriam, it's for your own safety that I don't want you to come with me; the roads heading to the oil fields are icy. Often Caterpillar tractors are placed along these trails to get the vehicles out from the ditches. We drive through frozen lakes to get to the rigs. I just don't want you to take any of those risks." John tried to make me understand his point, but he just added more fuel to my fire. I now knew all the hazardous stuff he dealt with everyday; drive through frozen lakes, picture it, what if the ice fractured?

Taking the bull by the horns this time I told my husband, "Honey, I'm not staying here one more day without you. I will feel a lot better if I'm with you in any circumstances than to be left alone again. Please understand, take me with you or send me back to my parents!" He knew I was serious and had no choice but to accept my request. I then had the opportunity to know my husband more, and learned the adventurous spirit he had.

Our decision created a bit of a conflict among some of John's colleagues. When the other engineers saw I accompanied my husband on his trips to the oil well-sites, I heard them criticize him, "Are you stupid or what John? You can't bring your wife to these forsaken places. Don't you realize the dangers you are putting her through?" This time I understood every word they said and furiously in half English, half Spanish I'd butt in, "My husband not tiene *culpa caramba;* it's me that wants to come. If not *prohibido,* I keep on coming; no *me importa* if is not right by you."

My husband, choking with laughter and hugging me, explained, "You have presented your case very well." I thought so too! I suppose John later explained more to his colleagues, because never again did they meddle in my coming or going. On the contrary they were always friendly and respectful. My husband and I became used to the companionship of our trips together and I had the opportunity to live in diverse and beautiful places that I otherwise would have never seen.

It was now September and my senses were filled with the scenic beauty. The sight and scent impacted me as John and I drove through the dazzling multicolored forest of the fall in Alberta. Every tree, every branch seemed to be speaking and singing an *Alleluia* to life. In Bolivia we didn't have the four seasons of the year so well defined. So never before I had experienced nature's awesomeness and magnificence, like now in Canada.

Perhaps everything was overblown because I carried within me the fruit of our love, and John now knew. Main reason, we were on our way to Calgary; coming out from the backcountry, oil fields, forest and bears. I had covered a lot of territory in Alberta as well as British Columbia; my experiences of the last six months had been more than just geographically instructive.

Going back to civilization was certainly good, getting to see John's people again was a bonus and getting everything ready for the birth of our baby an odyssey ahead. We had not one stitch of furniture or a cozy nest to come to, but in the next few days we got it all.

Once we settled in, I went in search for a Catholic parish. I still needed a link to compensate what I had left behind: my parents and friends. Soon I struck gold, the parish priest, Fr. Nicola, who I learned had a mixture of Polish and Italian blood running through his veins, the minute he open his mouth conquered my heart.

Out of the many attributes that the priest had that he spoke Spanish fluently was the best! Most of his pastoral life was performed in South American countries, in Argentina the longest; therefore he understood my culture well as it was similar.

John also bonded with Fr. Nicola. Our new friend didn't need a formal invitation to come and see us. He was always welcome in our home. Nicola would just show up at our front door, a bottle of wine in one hand for John and a bouquet of flowers in the other for me, loudly saying, "*Hola* is anyone home?" I believe he even appreciated my cooking; it had gotten better by then!

Hours before our son decided to make an early entrance into this world, I tirelessly worked on a thorough house cleaning. It was as if *Mr. Clean* himself inspired me. I washed and cleaned everything that got in my way, from floors, to ceilings, to walls, to every corner and every square inch of the nine hundred square foot apartment, I attacked it. With plenty of time before John came home, I even ironed some of his clothes and cooked one of his favorite dishes. My hard day's work ended with a fabulous splash in the tub and then I prettied myself for my husband's return from his office.

"Perhaps I have eaten a little too much," I thought, when around 11:30 pm, an uncomfortable stomach pain woke me up. Our baby was not due for at least two more weeks, so I didn't relate the pains I was experiencing to my pregnancy. Instead, I continued to believe my discomfort was a mere indigestion. Finally, at about 1:00 am, my water broke and realized I was going into labor; without any delay I woke John up.

Nervously he tried to get dressed. If it were not for the pain that came in flashes, I would have just sat laughing at his efforts. He first put both of his legs in one of the pants' legs, then took off his pants and tried again. His nervousness increased, this time the zipper turned out in the back. John finally managed to get dressed. As we were leaving the house, he remembered to call my doctor. The phone rang and rang and to his despair he only got the answering service. Impatiently I heard him nervously said, "My wife is in labor. I need someone to get a hold of Dr. Brown. We're on our way to the hospital."

It was only the beginning of November and winter had already begun. It had snowed on and off for the entire week, which made roads and streets very slippery. No big deal, my husband was one of the ones born with the expertise of driving well in icy conditions. He got us safely to the hospital.

An unconcerned woman behind the reception desk, coldly responded to my husband's inquires for Dr. Brown, "He is out of town, away on holidays," Not a good start. Doctor Brown was the person who was supposed to deliver my baby and he was away! It was unforeseen circumstance, true; our little one was not expected to arrive for at least two more weeks.

Still, it was upsetting. He was the doctor I had learned to trust and now someone else was paged; a complete stranger took his place! Totally stressed, I was wheeled to the delivery area, where my husband was not even allowed to be with me. A silly guideline protected men from being by their wives' sides through the labor pains. Instead they smoked cigars in the waiting room to calm their stress, ha-ha.

I certainly didn't feel like laughing much at that specific moment. On the contrary, I felt deserted, ugly, and in horrendous pain. I needed my mother next to me, but she was thousands of miles away and still not having a full command of the English language didn't help matters. To top it off, a woman not too sympathetic who acted more like a jailer than a nurse was in charge of preparing me.

At one point, when my frustration and pain reached the extreme and I started to cry, she ruthlessly gave me a slap in the face and said, "Don't be hysterical." I thought these things only took place in thriller movies, but it actually happened. Stunned, I stopped crying. I suppose the slap helped.

Later I was amazed at how much physical pain I had been able to endure while in delivery; more remarkable yet how easily all was forgotten after my baby was born. "It's a boy," the doctor said. While still carrying the baby, I had prayed for a girl, thinking the great companion she would be in her Dad's absences. Yet now that I held the little bundle of flesh close to my heart, I could not be any happier. I was a mother of a boy now! My yen from before did not exist anymore. I was excited, ecstatic; none of those words came even close to explain my joy!

Only then I mentioned to John the trick the unplanned wedding date had played on us. He was thrilled it happened! Then to make him laugh about dates I told him, "Good thing we are not back home. Imagined the amusing time all the little old ladies will have, counting with their fingers how many months went by, trying to figure if we'd had our fun before our wedding or not." They'd be unaware of the complexity of everything or that our baby was actually two weeks premature, but such was life back in my hometown.

John and I were pompous parents, but our inexperience was as obvious as our love; a day or two after our baby and I were released from the hospital, my husband and I decided to give our son his first bath at home. If the little fellow could only speak as he saw us preparing his bath, he would have said, "Hey Mom, Dad, guys what do you think you are doing?"

Pillows were set on the hard wood floor bellow the baby's tub in case his little soapy body would slip through our hands. The bubble bath directions went unread, the water temperature was not closely checked, but through trial and error we gradually learned and fortunately our baby survived our parental unawareness

Naturally our son had to be baptized, so we asked Fr. Nicola to christen him. John had no problem with the names I chose: John, Paul, William. The first after him, Paul was the name I liked best and coincidentally together with John, made an ideal combination; William was after my father. As the water was poured on our son's little head, we heard Nicola say, "I baptize thee with the name of John, Paul, William, and Peter Arthur, in the Name of the Father, and of the Son, and of the Holy Ghost. He had added Peter to the string of names our baby already carried. My husband and I looked at each other inquisitively, but waited; we could not inquire about the glitch in the middle of the ceremony.

At the end our curiosity was satisfied, "Nicola, did you make a mistake, or did you think our son didn't have enough names?" John asked. His usual big smile broadened, as our friend humorously explained, "Oops! You must forgive me; I must admit I got carried away. I figured John Paul William could be blessed with a name of my own choosing and the Apostle Peter's name fitted perfectly well." He chuckled loudly as he ended his speech.

It was this way that our son began his little life armored and blessed by all those names, but for us, he was just John Paul; John *Paulito* for me.

After his birth I never felt lonely again, nor frightened if my husband was detained somewhere by his work. I now had my baby as my companion. I had someone else besides my husband to love and care for. My life was complete!

Every so often I chose to continue with the trips with my husband, our son roaming together with us. No hotel reservations ahead of time, we just took what ever the destination-town had to offer for our lodging. John Paulito who accommodated easily to all circumstances had no problem sleeping on beds other than his, but he absolutely hated sharing his sleeping spot with anyone, not even with Mom. He would fuss and kick until the bed was all to himself.

Most lodgings provided baby cribs, or cots, except for this particular hotel where it had neither. Past his bedtime, our nine-month-old son, a little cranky needed to have his own bed and our room had only a queen size one. He would have been happy to have it all for himself, however that was not going to happen. To control the situation John and I crammed the tub in the bathroom with extra pillows, blankets and made it like a cozy crib. Thankfully John Paulito graciously accepted the innovation; otherwise his father and I might have ended up using it ourselves. Actually J. P. loved it! Never a dull moment

Except that with the good came the bad. This time, with the car packed to the rim we headed for Peace River, a town in northern B.C where John's presence was required for a longer period of time. My husband's company had rented a large unit in a Motel that even had a kitchenette to give us some comfort with our stay. Certainly John Paul and I were included in the plan.

One evening, John was called to tend problems at a well site and had to leave, but not before he instructed me to keep the door locked. "After all we are in unknown territory Myriam, and one can't be careful enough." He said smiling and giving us a kiss he left.

An hour or two later all hell broke loose. The fellows who occupied the unit next to ours tried to pry our door open; drunk as skunks shouting obscenities; I heard one of them clearly say, "Hey little woman, come out and have some fun with us. We will show you our p... you will really have a good time with us." Likely they were aware that my husband was not around, even in their stupor.

Petrified by their harassment I softly held John Paul in my arms and tenderly told him, "Be quiet, John Paulito. I'm afraid. Those men might hurt us; we need to be silent as little mice until your father gets back, okay?" J. P. kept quiet. I suppose our silence convinced the men that no one was around, though a few minutes later, once more someone tried to force their way in. I didn't dare move!

Through the 20 months John and I had been married, what impressed me the most about my husband was his good nature and friendly disposition. Yet, when he came back that night and learned what happened, I saw the other side of my loving husband, and his reaction scared me!

John grabbed his gun; a while back I'd learned it was quite normal to have one in the car or at home for self-protection. Of course I knew John had them, as well as several hunting guns, but I had never seen him use them other than on target or hunting practices; but now blinded with anger my husband went out.

Our son was already fast asleep. So out of frightened curiosity or foolishness I followed him and saw John kick the next-door unit wide open, and pointing his gun to the drunkards, who with the noisy impact had aroused from their alcoholic lethargy, bellowed at them, "Get your butts up. You are leaving town immediately, unless you want to die!"

The arrival of the RCMP, called by the caretaker, brought the situation to a standstill. John informed them of the intended assault on his wife and child. The officers understanding the situation reinforced my husband's ultimatum saying, "You will come with us now, and tomorrow when you all sober up you will leave town."

The next day, after a fine was paid, they left. My husband who also reported the incident to his superiors demanded back up from them, "These sons of b...have harassed my wife. I don't want to see them ever again in town while I'm here, or I'll resign." In much need of John's expertise his boss made the necessary arrangements with the other company, as well as with the police to have those men removed from the area.

A notable point in my life, it convinced me more than ever that I not only had married an incredible prince charming, but also a good provider and again a gallant and well armed warrior ready to protect his wife and son!

It seems that John always had a new card under his hat, he never stop surprising me. One day, once we were back in Calgary, out of the blue told me, "Honey, I'm bored stiff. I want to see other parts of the world. I need to do something else, have new experiences and share them with you and our son."

Not quite thirty years old, it was his impulsive and adventurous spirit taking over. I would soon learn that this facet happened to be the highlight of his personality. So quietly I listened to the rest of his oratory, "I'll look for another job. I don't know where, but something good I'm sure will come up." He closed his speech with a kiss and a huge smile. I then remembered his words when we were just married "Don't worry dear. I'll show you the world."

No sooner said than it was done. An Australian company's advertisement in the local newspapers attracted my husband's attention; "We are in need of a Geological Engineer for our operations in Australia. The individual should have extensive knowledge in all aspects of exploration, as well as experience in the exploitation of oil fields; the best applicant will be well remunerated." Exactly what John had in mind! The description fitted my husband's skills like a glove. He applied for the job and on return mail my husband's dream came to be a reality.

In fact A. B. Robertson & Associates wanted John in Melbourne as soon as possible and were willing to pay for all expenses, including for John Paul and myself. This happened in the later part of 1961.

Frankly I was not impressed with the idea. Australia was farther away from my childhood home; this time even an ocean would separate me from my family in South America. John, who really wanted to go, played a trump card. He enticed me with exciting promises, "Darling, before we go to Australia, I'll take you to visit your parents. John Paul will get to meet his grandparents and we'll all have a grand time." How could I resist such an offer? I accepted.

In the end the plan didn't work out as planned. Unfinished work in Calgary and my husband's imminent duties in Australia prevented him from coming along with us.

It was undoubtedly a difficult journey on my own; our son was a very active one year old child. John Paulito, who started to walk when he was just eight months old, was now a speedy runner and a better climber; he got up on top of chairs and counters like a pro. Our son had proven many times over that he feared nothing.

Even so I was not about to lose the opportunity to see my parents again, no matter how trying my little angel could be on the trip. Moreover, aside from his acrobatic skills, J.P. was actually an adorable child, not the least spoiled or shy. Any female from age two to 84, who came near him became captive by his cute smile, his olive green eyes, and his blond hair; they were excellent points in his favor.

With mixed feelings, happy and sad, I said good-bye to my husband, not intimidated any longer by the long journey ahead.

John necessarily had to give me some words of advice, "Darling, I know you'll be cautious and watchful over our son. However I'll say it again, be very careful and please don't talk to strangers."

He looked worry and I felt I had to reassure him, "I promise. I won't talk to strangers, especially the male ones...right dear?" I said laughing knowing my husband's protectiveness.

Last kisses and John Paul and I boarded the plane. Via San Francisco, Miami, Lima, La Paz, and our last touch down Cochabamba. The itinerary was hard enough for anyone, let alone for me with my toddler. In San Francisco some passengers disembarked, the rest the same as us, continued in the same plane to Florida. All had gone well until then, but no sooner we had landed in Miami, the excitement began.

It was impossible to contain my child; he ran everywhere. I suppose he had to release his energy after the many hours of being restrained. The aircraft was beautiful, the flight attendants excellent, but for my little one it was just a large cage where he had to behave well. Now he had open spaces to explore and as we were passing through Immigration, I got distracted for seconds and he took the opportunity to escape!

Nowhere to be seen, I panicked; he was so little, anyone could grab my son and disappear. I called out his name, some travelers on the same flight, who already knew him, came to my aid and went looking for J. P. He was not far; the rascal had been hiding behind some large suitcases, giggling. After the scare I didn't know if to scold my child or embrace him; I did both.

I didn't want to risk having a similar situation again; so with some time in my hands before our next flight to Lima, I searched, found and bought a child's harness. The most suitable control for my son, none of the persons who helped me before came along and while I tended to passports and luggage John Paul was attach to my waist.

Upon arrival in Lima I only had time to disembark from Pan-Am, get the suitcases through Custom's and embark them on LAB, the Bolivian airline. I barely had chance to say hello to my sister and Raul, who waited for us at the airport; embraced them and say good-bye. In between all the hassle, John Paulito was either in my arms or attached to me with his new umbilical cord. I was not taking any more chances!

When we arrived in Cochabamba, I was exhausted. Not my son, who had his regular naps and snacks; he was as fresh as green lettuce, and now ready to have some more fun. What a relief to be greeted by my parents. Better yet, when my father ecstatic over meeting his grandson took over the management, not aware of what he was getting into!

John Paul, overjoyed, conducted himself as though he had known his Grandpa from the beginning of his little life and my father was also entrapped by his grandson's charm. While me, I was delighted to be a daughter again and what a treat to be liberated of my regular mothering and household duties!

Customarily around 11am, father enjoyed going for a stroll. Impeccably dressed he walked to the main *plaza*, about four blocks from our home, the meeting place with some of his friends. Retired army fellows like him, who served under him during the four-year Chaco war; warfare between Bolivia and Paraguay. Dad now incorporated John Paulito on these promenades. J. P. dressed in his best clothes, bow tie included; they both looked like a million dollars taking the stroll in the later part of the morning.

It was something special to watch this honorable grey-haired gentleman walk with this well-dressed wee toddler, no more than two and a half feet tall; tightly holding one of his grandfather's fingers as they marched towards la plaza, and because he was Guillermo's grandson, he was also befriended by these courageous men.

From la plaza they continued to the Social Club, where father enjoyed reading international newspapers; he smoked a cigar or two or played pool while J.P. enjoyed a creamy ice cream. He liked the attention he was receiving, but more than anything he loved to be with his grandpa; I was also having a grand time with my family and friends.

Over a month had gone by when father decided, "We'll all go to Lima next week. I want to visit Vicky and her family. I want to include them in our happiness; this could pretty much be my last chance to be reunited with both my daughters and their families. I know John will not be joining us, but there isn't much we can do about it."

Of course my mother and I were just as excited as him. Dad's idea was grand. Vicky and her husband were also thrilled; both greeted us with open arms. Sandra and Sergio, their two children, and John Paul got along splendidly. It was at this first meeting that the boys bonded for life; their birthdays in October and November were only 20 days apart. They played and got into mischief together but were closely watched by the two nannies my sister had in her service.

Soon country clubs, beaches and yachts, plus eating all the Peruvian food I could eat (the yummy *seviches,* followed by pisco sours, *anticuchos,* or *papas a la wankaina,* together with some *Cuba Libres)* got all my attention. Distracted by the grand time I was having, I shut my eyes to the fact that close to two months had gone by since I said good-bye to my husband, and avoided thinking that it was time for me to join him again.

At first John patiently wrote, "Sweetheart, I'm very lonely. I need you both here with me." The second month came and went and in his sixth letter, my husband began to show his displeasure over our extended absence. In the last one I received, completely annoyed he wrote, "You better get back to me now, or don't bother coming back at all."

An ultimatum all right! Similar to the one he posed before we got married. I knew he meant it. So I packed up, bade farewell to my family and flew with our son back to John. He left me no other choice; I had to obey!

On the flight to Australia, John Paul behaved exceptionally well. The journey had less transfers, and the enticement of seeing his Dad again was likely what did it; besides I had threatened him with the old stand by saying, "I'll tell your father if you misbehave and probably he won't be too happy with you." The threat seemed to have worked and the plane landed safely in Sydney.

Within seconds John Paul and I were in John's arms; he had been waiting for us at the gate's terminal and for a short moment we became the airport's main attraction!

EARLY JULY, 1985

NO MORE THAN FOUR DAYS WENT BY AND I HAD FOUND JIM. IN MY troubled mind I had even considered that God himself intervened in my hunt.

So the minute we met, I straightforwardly asked him, "Jim do you have any connections in the cocaine trade?" His facial expression changed; turning pale he frowned and kept silent. I realized I had been too abrupt. Surely he feared to be implicated in an illegal activity and obviously he was not about to provide me with any help or information.

"No. I don't know anyone. Since I was released from prison, I haven't touched the stuff," he strongly stated but avoided eye contact with me. Sensing he was not telling the truth, I changed my approach and gently pleaded with him, "I swear to you, I'm not working for the police. The truth is Jim that I have a big problem. I need a large amount of money quickly and I don't have a chance in obtaining it legally. You are the only one I know. Please help me."

Perhaps because of the assistance John and I had provided him in the past, Jim opened up and ultimately agreed to come to my aid. "I'll call you back. I'll see what I can come up with. I'll let you know.

The next Thursday, Jim called inviting me to come to his place and meet a couple of his friends. Actually, they were his business associates. After the introductions Jim explained, "José here is Bolivian, and he is the expert in preparing the drug. Bernard is from Yugoslavia. He handles the deals, has connections in Brazil and Spain." Blinded by my despair, I didn't consider I was now entering into the shadowy part of the underworld. Instead, with great relief I only saw three clean-cut young men who were willing to help me!

Jim then proceeded to explain the business aspects for the transactions, "We don't have an operating capital, and so we need to get 50% of the money paid up front for the orders. The remaining balance must be paid in full once the product is ready and in your hands."

Bernard, who seemed to be the one more versed in the particulars, took over saying, "Our price for each gram of cocaine is seven American dollars, but you can be certain that the drug will be 99% pure." The Yugoslavian produced a calculator from his pocket and punching some figures, he added, "The merchandise prepared by us can easily be sold in Brazil for eighteen American dollars. If you go a little bit further, like let's say Spain, you can get twice that price."

This information, plus what I had learned about what car merchants obtained in a deal, matched. There was a good profit margin potential in the trade; exactly what I needed. The rumors were now facts. Before leaving I assured them, "The minute I'm organized and have the money, I'll let you know. By the way, how much time do you need to prepare the drug?"

Bernard hands moving and waving about while talking, answered, "Oh, I would say a week or a week and a half more or less." Happy with the result of my inquest, I thanked them, shook their hands, and left.

In only one interview I had all the facts and figures. I trusted these men immediately. I didn't even consider the possibility that once I handed over the money they could just walk away with it, leaving me empty handed. After all what did I know about them? I was just happy that part of my quest was partly completed

George's suggestions and my recent inquiries about Paris settled where John Paul should go, but there were still many unanswered questions. The possibility to do more over the phone was nil, so I decided it was best if John Paul went to France to investigate and obtain the information himself.

Even if the treatment didn't come right away, at least we would have a better idea of what we needed to do next. I could not just sit idle; something had to be done before it was too late, even if it was an expensive way to do it. Eager for immediate results I didn't even see the futility of such a hectic trip. I ran on pure adrenaline. My rational mind was out of control and if an obstacle jumped at me, I found instant solutions.

As it happened, when I realized that John Paul might need some kind of support over in France, it is then I remembered Judith. Married to a French engineer, she presently lived in Cannes; it was a distance away from Paris, but close enough. We were not blood related but we considered ourselves cousins. Her father and my father had been the best of friends, so close that from childhood they were taken for brothers. I knew I could count on Judith; I was sure she could be of assistance if J. P.'s presence in France was longer than expected.

A freelance tour guide, my surrogate cousin visited her father in La Paz twice a year and in order to supplement her visits, she traded in artisan Bolivian goods. I had often acted as her buyer and shipper; this kept us in contact. When we last spoke she had mentioned, "I plan to be in La Paz mid September. I'll let you know the exact date later. I'll place my order for the crafts I need then."

I had to act quickly to check on her availability; I still had a good chance to catch her at home. My call went through and Judith answered, "Hi, how are you?" she said recognizing my voice. "Is everything okay down there? she asked and without waiting for my reply inquired again, "Are you calling to find out the date I plan to come?"

It was my turn to speak, "We are all well thanks, and no, I'm not calling you about your trip, I know it's in September." I certainly didn't want anyone to know of my son's illness, not even Judith. So directly I told the story I prepared for her. "John Paul has a field trip programmed through his university, to go to Paris. It will happen in the next few days. I believe he might have some free time to visit your area. Would you mind hosting him for a short time?"

"I'd love to have John Paul. I have a spare bedroom. He is welcome to come any time," Judith happily responded. While she was still speaking, my brain furiously spinning had another brilliant idea; what if I asked Judith to help me find a buyer for the merchandise?

Calmly but with a note of excitement in my voice I told her, "I'm going to start a new business, Judith. It will probably involve me going to France in the next little while. I have the feeling it might interest you. It's a great way to make good money." My overture seemed to create a certain amount of curiosity. She wanted to know the particulars; in a few seconds my brain had concocted a plan that could fit well with Judith's forthcoming trip.

"You know me well Myriam. I'm always looking for ways to make extra money. Tell me what it is all about and maybe we can work together?" Judith responded laughing loudly.

"It's too long to explain over the phone. I'll tell you what; I'll send you a letter with all the details. I'll ask John Paul to take it for me if he stops to see you, otherwise he will just mail it to you. Mind you, he doesn't know beans about what I planned to do, so don't bother asking him anything. If you like what I have to offer, you can let me know when I call you next time. Okay?"

I had good reasons for turning to Judith and include her in my plan. I knew she was experiencing financial difficulties after the purchase of their new home. A good portion of their income went to pay the mortgage payments and her visits to her Dad became less viable. If my idea was accepted, she could easily resume those trips, but the main reason was because Judith was a part of the fashionable society in Cannes. I fancied that she might know people with status who occasionally used cocaine.

Introduced by a couple of friends in the crowd John and I now frequented, we had experimented with the stuff. The drug was effective, particularly if the alcohol intake had been excessive; the impairment dissipated almost immediately. Logically I assumed now that it had to be a common practice in Cannes. It would be then easy for Judith to find someone who in turn might know someone else with contacts in these types of dealings.

As soon I hung up the phone, I booked a flight for John Paul on credit, the return date open. Long time customers, the travel agency had no need to worry; the debt would be in American dollars anyway, therefore protected against the rampant inflation. Once everything was in place I told my son, who was not aware of what I had in mind. "John Paul, you are going to France next Friday. I believe George's suggestion is sound. You shall seek medical help in Paris."

John Paul looked at me as if I had gone insane. He was somewhat conscious of our economic situation, but before he could say anything I continued, "I wish I could give you more concrete information prior to your trip, but there isn't much we can do from this end. While in France it will be up to you to find out all you can: the cost and the time frame for the treatment."

How little did I know about the terrifying illness to expect it could be treated as a common malady? Some of my brain cells must have died with the pain, but what propelled my frenzy the most was that John Paul's health didn't seem yet compromised by the ill effects of the infirmity; therefore I had to hurry while there was still hope.

To ease my son's concern I added, "Remember Judith? She lives in Cannes. I spoke with her and she'll be happy to lodge you if you need to stay in France for a while. You could take the train or a bus from Paris; I understand the prices are very reasonable.

You will take some money and I'll wire more as soon as you let me know the cost for the treatment."

At first my son didn't want to go. He didn't want to exacerbate our financial situation. Artfully, I reassured him that money was no object. J.P. had no reason not to believe me. He knew I was the one who handled the family and factory's finances and agreed to go. Naturally I explained to him the fabricated tale I created for Judith's benefit. To simplify matters I asked J.P. to maintain the same story for his Dad and everyone else's sake.

Elaborating around the school trip tale, I told John, close family members and friends that John Paul was going to France. Everyone was happy for J.P while my heart ached, but I figured that if John had to be in the dark about our son's illness, the less he knew of my future plans the better off we would all be.

The amount of money I would need to cover John Paul's initial medical bills was still in a question mark, but the thirty to forty thousand dollars figure, given to us during John's episode with cancer, became a good reference point. Surely John Paul's treatment shouldn't be too lengthy; therefore I had no long-term trepidations. My concern was to obtain the thirty thousand dollars, and if necessary later obtain more. So with more guesswork than knowledge, I wrote the letter to Judith explaining my business proposition.

Dear Judith

I hope Jean Pierre and the children are fine. I wish I could tell you the same about us, but it is not so. A while back I told you John had a serious operation, remember? But I never mentioned that a cancerous growth was removed from his bladder. Unfortunately once cancer strikes it lingers over you like a shadow and with the political and economical unrest happing in our country, I worry. Because presently we don't have the means to undertake any expenses related to treatments, operations etcetera.

I'm sure you are aware of all the political chaos and economical catastrophe our country is going through. As a result everyone around here is having hardships, including us. In view of all this, I'm investigating a way to make money. I don't want to shock you with what I'm about to tell you; just keep an open mind okay?

It has to do with cocaine. People here buy the stuff at very low cost and resale high. These types of deals are wide spread in our country. Families are turning to this trade to cope with the economical difficulties; I decided to join in and I need your help to find someone interested in buying it. You probably know people with money in Cannes. Likely some already use the drug in their parties, to sober up.

Remember when Jean Pierre and you visited us a while back? We all drank a bit too much and Jean Pierre and John sniffed the stuff and immediately composed themselves?

Getting straight to the point, what I need from you is to find a contact among those people. Someone interested in making extra money and you will get a percentage of the profit as a commission for your effort too. How does it sound?

If you are interested, start looking. Just say yes, when I call you later in the month. If you are not, forget everything I told you and make sure you destroy this letter. I wouldn't want strange hands getting hold of it, okay?

Furthermore, it's best we refer to the drug as the "stuff," or "la cosa," when we are talking about it over the phone. We need to be careful. Well that is all for now Judith, looking forward to the next time we talk.

In the meantime say hello to Jean Pierre and the kids.

Love Myriam

Australia, 1962

JOHN WAS IMMEDIATELY PUT IN CHARGE OF THE EXPLORATION and exploitation of oil wells that the company, Robertson and Associates had on the go. My husband felt like a fish in water. This is what he loved, but just as before, his work took him away from home, this time to different regions of Australia.

Occasionally John Paul and I would join him, but not too often. Not familiar with the surroundings or accommodations available my husband didn't want us to take any chances. "You are safer and better off if you remain at home. Besides I don't know how the bosses would appreciate a woman's intrusion in the work field," he said and I accepted. My maternity and the travels with my husband seemed to have forged my character, it was now almost fully developed, and so I didn't need to be my husband's shadow as much any more.

The company had rented for us a large as well as comfortable house in Sandringham. A bayside residential suburb, 18 km south from Melbourne's city centre, two hundred meters from the oceanfront and from a beautiful golden beach, surely splendid in the summer. The brick dwelling had four bedrooms, two would have been more than enough for us, but it was their choice and they paid the rent. It had hardwood floors throughout, including the living and dining room, with wood-burning fireplaces in all; central heating was a rare commodity in these types of houses.

Melbourne's climate was not the best during the winter season; it rained almost every day and it was said that the same happened in fall as well as part of spring. No wonder there was a need for so many fireplaces; to keep the house warm we had them all burning 24/7. After all the company also picked up the tab for the firewood use. Often confined in the house because of the precipitation, the dwelling supplied an exciting amusement for our son, who was now a year and a half old.

John Paul loved to play hide and seek in this big great house. He would run and hide somewhere and say, *"Come Mommy, fin' me."* His greatest delight was when I said, "John Paulito, where are you honey? I can't find you!" He giggled but didn't answer. Pretending I didn't hear his laughter, I called again, "Come on honey, you are scaring Mommy." He then would come out from hiding with his little arms up, saying, "Ere 'am Mommy, 'ere." He actually spoke well; only some letters of the alphabet were left out from his words.

We had comfort and beauty; nonetheless a bit tedious without the participation of the key member of the team, so everything was always better when John was with us. When he was around, the three of us dressed to kill went on exploratory trips. One of our favorites was the scenic route to Melbourne, on the Sandringham Railway Line; once in downtown we strolled around top of Collins Street, an incredibly affluent area. Multimillion-dollar corporations operated here, including Robertson and Associates, John's work place when he was not in the field. We blended well in that crowd and enjoyed it every bit!

Other times we took the City Circle Tram, which gave us the chance to glance and admire the Victorian and Gothic architecture prevailing in the core of Melbourne, such as St. Paul's Cathedral on Flinders St; an incredible sight to see. Yet we could not extend these trips for too long, John Paulito was with us and though he behaved well, at some point all was just too boring for him, which was acceptable since he was not quite two.

Summer brought an altogether different story. The past season was forgotten as our bodies began to store vitamin D; we let the bright sun brown our pale skin. Normally John was home on the weekends and with him around were extra special; loaded with food, drinks, towels, shovels, pails, and the like, the Arthur family headed for the beach.

First in one foot of water, then up to our knees and further up, we let the water of the Pacific Ocean cover our bodies, J.P. on John's shoulders. Swimming was fun though scary at times because of the sharks, but we soon learned to trust the aviators who in small planes made it safe for the wet masses. They circled the beaches and if a shark was sighted, the pilots immediately radioed the local stations. The warning devices installed around the beaches, were sounded and everyone in the water was out in a matter of seconds.

The fad continued to some evenings too. John Paulito and I waited for his father to return from work, with a basket of goodies; the plan was to eat supper at the beach. The minute J. P. saw his Dad, he hollered, "come daddy hurry up, let-go!" John, happy to please his son, hurried.

Habitually we swam until the night was well set; by then the water looked like a sea of black ink. Sharks were of some concern; no aviators or sirens to call us to safety around at this time, but our Australian neighbors, who seemed to know what they were doing, swam. Encouraged by their bravery, as good copycats we just followed their example, always on the look out for fins.

Being an outdoor family, if beaches were not in the plan, we went to a park in our neighborhood instead. Full of swings, merry-go-rounds and further away even a swimming pool; these were all perfect ways to entertain our son. John Paul, daring as always, kept his Dad and I on high alert. He loved to run to the other end of the pool and from where he would shout, "Mommy,

Daddy, look!" and purposely jump into the deep end, ignoring the danger.

His Dad had no choice but to immediately dive after him and pulled him to the surface, while I remain paralyzed with the dread that John Paulito could drown. It was not the case, never was; our son simply grinned at his mischief. He thus learned to swim at a very early age.

John because of his work often traveled to other Australian states, such as Queensland, South Australia, New South Wales, and Victoria. At Sale he took a major part in the discovery of the second most important oil field in the country; everyone in the company was elated. His future with the group could not be better, yet after the first year, when he was offered to renew his contract for an indefinite time, my husband declined. The decision was John's own. I didn't influence him, but perhaps he had sensed that Australia was not the country where I wanted to settle in permanently.

An important element was missing in our lives: friendships. No matter how hard we tried, the aloofness we found in Melbourne was unbreakable; the barrier of the culture was there. What's more I never stop feeling like a captive in Australia, perhaps a kind of phobia, after all in my eyes the entire continent no matter how large, was just an enormous island encircled by the ocean's immensity.

Even so, I would have never contradicted my husband had he chosen to stay. Probably John's decision came more because the enchantment of the adventure ended, crowned by the oil discovery. I didn't ask. I was just thrilled we were leaving the place.

On our flight back to California we had a few hours stopover at Nandi airport in Viti Levu, one of the main Fijian islands. As we walked to the airport's terminal, a warm and somewhat humid climate embraced us, and a diversity of exotic plants and palm trees, an incredibly beautiful sight welcomed us. In seconds, my husband and I fell in love with the place and John enthusiastically said, "We need to see it all. If it's possible, we should stay here for a few days."

Action followed his words. At the airline's stand, handing over our tickets to the teller John said, "We would like to change our itinerary and stay here for about a week, instead of just the hours specified in our tickets. Can this be arranged?" John's zeal was contagious, so the attendant responded in a similar manner, "Of course Mr. Arthur; we'd love to oblige you. By the way your flight has another stop in Hawaii; if you wish, it can also be prolonged?" My husband instinctively looked at me, but didn't say anything; he just answered, "Yes that will be great, please get it done!"

The young man got on the phone and the changes were accepted. Handing back our tickets he added, "We have a fantastic resort at the other side of the island called Cora Levu, accessed only by car." John attentively listened and with a mischievous look on his face, so common to him when something exciting was about to happen, said to the clerk, "We are going there; call us a taxi please."

Looking back at me said, "We'll have a second honeymoon darling; you are going to love it and John Paul too." Of course I loved it and rewarded my husband with a kiss, and a new adventure began, this time in paradise.

I had never before seen such exotic vegetation; the thought that we had landed in paradise was reinforced when we arrived at the hotel, a five star hotel complex. We chose one of the huts as our abode, rustic from outside, palm branches for roof, but inside the cabin was refined, hardwood floors throughout except for the bathroom, where marble predominated; not too far from the main building and only a few meters from the crystal-clear waters of the Pacific Ocean.

The place, the whole area was surrounded by verdant palm trees, ferns and orchids, all beyond one's imagination, the fragrance emanating was a gift to our nostrils; it was a dream come true and then there was the food. Seafood buffets were set everywhere with lobsters, humongous oysters, shrimp, exotic fruits, in addition to the excellent meals we ate at the hotel's chic dining room.

The swimming and playing around saved our waistlines; we did nothing but eat, sleep, swim and have fun. It was great! John Paul not quite two and a half years old tried everything; if he didn't like it, he spat the food saying, *"Excuse me! Yuck! I don't like it."* Yet, he continued experimenting and trying new things.

The hotel provided extraordinary childcare service. 6'8" male natives, well trained and gifted with the friendliest disposition occupied the post. Their black jet complexion and height didn't frighten John Paul; on the contrary he enjoyed being under the care of these unique nannies.

As a result, our evenings were also action-packed. John and I attended Fijian ethnic dance performances, or went dancing at one of the nearby clubs. Others we just had a romantic evening by the beach, with a glass of Pinot Noir or Champagne in our hands, sure that our little one was well taken care. It was hard to leave this enchanting island.

We still had Hawaii, our next sojourn, which could easily drain my husband's savings from Australia; the island apparently was on the expensive side to say the least. Yet John as usual had a positive remark, "Oh, nothing to worry about dear! We are young and an opportunity like this is hard to come by, besides I'll earn more money when we get home."

What could I have said? No? Of course not. I loved his idea. Besides it was his money; he had worked hard for it and living in the moment was as natural as breathing. We stayed and never regretted it. At the Waikiki beaches we saw old folks playing and having fun the same as us, but it felt good to be young!

Our final touchdown was in Los Angeles, California. Here the man I married, to whom I was still trying to adjust, with his best smile ever, the one he usually used when he wanted me to agree with him, said, "Honey, we'll stay here for a short time. I need to do some research before we continue to Canada."

I quietly listened, not understanding much of what he was now brewing. "I'm a Geological Engineer and my work always has evolved around the oil industry. I now want to go back to school and obtain a petroleum engineering degree. The more I know, the better job opportunities I'll get." I had nothing to say except that I commended his idea and I admired my husband all the more for it.

The University of Southern California offered him the right curriculum, but some U.S. regulations postponed his registration for the following semester. In a sense this was good, the extra stretch would buy him the time to replenish his wallet. We had depleted our finances and the few dollars left, paid for two adult tickets and one child on the Greyhound bus to Calgary; the change we used to buy some of our nourishment on the way up.

We arrived in town, so broke that John's mother had to pay for the taxi. Embarrassed, I wanted to hide. Not my husband. He was not a bit concerned, certain to have in the next day or two a good job and money.

Again he was right. His old company in Calgary hired him back. His mom was treated to a lovely dinner for the money she paid for the taxi. Invited by our in-laws, we stayed at their home for the next six-months.

John worked arduously and made enough money to cover the university's tuition, school supplies, and meet other major expenses for the first semester. He was even able to purchase a 1958 Ford sedan, put into terrific condition by Gordon, his step dad who happened to be a mechanic. By then, our U.S. green cards arrived.

In the fall of 1963 we headed for Los Angeles; taking turns at the wheel, 32 hours later, triumphantly we arrived. We found a motel not too far from the university grounds and after a short rest and refreshing, with the help of a newspaper, our hunt for a place to call home began. I no longer was the naïve Bolivian girl John married almost four years ago; he was responsible for my change. I had become a Mom and through all the travels I gained confidence. Household chores, finances, and budgeting were now easy tasks and shared responsibility with my husband.

Two days later our search was rewarded; a housing complex ideally located, only three blocks from the university, had one unit for rent. Nine residences in total were built around a court-yard in a Californian-Spanish style that gave the place a cozy atmosphere. It was furnished and within our budget, however it needed an exhaustive makeover.

Before moving in, John sanded and re-finished the hardwood floors. I painted the walls, and cleaning the stove and bathroom fixtures we both sweated profusely until they became white again. The facelift brought the apartment closer to our standards. The brisk promenades John had to take heading for the university helped him developed stronger leg muscles, which in turn saved us gas money.

Our new habitat was almost perfect, except that the other residents didn't have small children. It was not the best setting for our child; there was only so much Mom could do to keep up with his bounciness. What John Paul needed was to have playmates.

Friends had been an important element in life. Back home I always had them, cousins too, but because of our constant travels, John Paul had neither. Los Angeles was our fixed point of residence for the next while; I had to find a way to amend the present situation.

John Paul and I went for walks around the neighborhood and discovered a park where we met a few moms; they had kids, boys and girls. Through them I learned of a daycare facility not two blocks away. Right away my son and I proceeded to check the place out, and found an amazingly enticing daycare center. The nursery, run by a handful of young Cuban nuns, was more than I ever dreamed existed: tiny desks and chairs in one room, small beds where the children had their naps in another, miniscule toilets and sinks in the bathroom. It seemed as we had entered a fairytale land.

John Paul jumping up and down immediately said, "Mommy, Mommy I want to stay and play here, please, please!!!" He had seen little ones playing around. The nun who had come to greet us answered all my queries, "Yes, our day nursery provides a safe haven for small children. Yes, we have an opening for your son. Yes, he will be fine here. The center opens at seven, the children need to be picked up no later than five and the fee is $20.00 dollars per week; lunch is included."

What a grand discovery; John Paul could now have friends. As for me, it opened a new possibility; from the moment John had decided to go back to school, my heartfelt desire was to work and be of some help with our financial needs. Except that I knew he had negative thoughts on the subject.

John brought up in the old school went by a well-rooted principle, "The man of the house should be the sole provider for his family." It was not going to be easy to convince him otherwise. Besides he would also challenge me, "Who do you think will look after our son? Do you want to leave John Paul with strangers?"

Now I had a good chance to persuade him. If I succeeded some of his time could be freed up. Encouraged by these thoughts I collected the nerve to talk to him, "John, you should let me work. After all I'm your wife and I want to help." I pleaded with him. The frown in my husband's forehead deepened as he stubbornly rebuked, "No, I don't like it. You should know this by now. I can manage fine without you having to work; I'll work weekends to earn extra money to cover all the expenses."

My stubborn streak flared up too; I didn't like to be given no for an answer. I had to win this battle, so subtly I counter-attacked, "Don't you see what is happening to our marriage, to John Paul? We don't have any quality time together anymore. You get up in the morning and off you go to the university for the entire day. At night you expect us to be quiet, so you can bury your head in your books. Now, you tell me you plan to work weekends too! When will you have time for me and for our son? He is so young. He desperately tries to get your attention and you don't even notice."

My observations seemed to have touched John's heart, because suddenly he said, "Okay, okay; I'll accept your idea, but you need to understand that before you set yourself off looking for work, I want your promise that our son will not be neglected. Secondly that the work you find has to be in a clean and decent environment." He didn't say it, but I gathered what he meant: no bars or nightclubs. He was still zealously protective. I understood his point and with a kiss we sealed the agreement.

In the later part of 1963, while entertaining John Paul at the park a delightful lady approached us smiling. There was nothing intimidating about her; she was almost my mother's age, very friendly but also seemed lonely.

Alice loved to go to concerts and as our friendship progressed, knowing I was in no position to afford this type of pursuit, she invited me to come along as her companion. John too, but occupied with his studies he declined the invitations. He watched over our son instead, who fortunately was already fast sleep.

Conversing with my new friend, I made her aware of my aspirations, "I want to work and help my husband with our finances; I'll be looking for work. I've taken businesses course, so I could handle office work. I was trained as a volunteer by the Red Cross and I assisted nurses at the general hospital in my city, but I have no references. Still I've got to try."

A day or two after, Alice with a fairy godmother look on her face said, "My doctor is in need of a medical assistant." She kept silent for seconds, wanting to give a soundless effect to her next words; I didn't dare interrupt. "Gloria, his current assistant is taking maternity leave. He needs someone to replace her. I know Harry is willing to accept a person with no experience; he will train the individual. Myriam, you are perfect for the job. You should apply. I'll tell Harry about you." Appreciative for her interest, I thanked Alice.

Upbeat by her words, I jumped at the opportunity and called Dr. H. Dunbar's office to set up an interview. Alice had spoken highly of me and the meeting went great! I could not believe my luck, Dr. Dunbar, a well-known family doctor in Beverly Hills, after a short meeting gave me the position. "You can start immediately; Gloria will train you before she leaves. Your working schedule will be from 9am 'til 5pm, with one hour break around 12.30," he said with a warm smile.

"Thank you Dr. Dunbar, I would love to work for you and I don't see any problem, but first I have to inform my husband. I'll let you know the minute I've done it, if this okay by you," I responded and went home happy and proud. The job would certainly match John's criteria.

It did, and when he learned I'd struck gold, he was happy for me.

Later on the same day, we went together to see Dr. Dunbar. After I introduced them, I said "I can start immediately, but would it be alright if I start Monday? In need still to make the arrangements with the daycare and establish a new schedule for John Paul.

My idea was a reality now. Of course the money I earned compared to what John would have brought working weekends was minimal, but it liberated his time, paid for the roof over our heads and food. In addition, my husband got some consulting assignments through the university and was well paid.

John completed his first semester. He then set himself in motion to make enough money for the next term; tuition and books were very costly. It was a cycle we agreed to go through until graduation date. Through the summer he worked as a roughneck on the oil rigs of Long Beach and San Pedro. My hero worked six-days per week for eight to sixteen hours per day and longer if necessary. He took shifts for others and accumulated double and triple pay, the money was exceptionally good, but involved hard labor and it was dangerous and dirty.

One only had to see him at the end of the day to understand how grimy! He came home covered in black oil from head to toes; laundromats didn't appreciate our business, no wonder. It was a mad race; money was the final objective. John had a goal in his mind and nothing stood in his way.

At the end of the three months my husband had made enough money to cover all of the university expenses, even purchased a second vehicle for our comings and goings. I also had great success in my new career, I quickly learned all the duties of an M.O.A, and became Dr. Dunbar's perfect assistant.

Even in all this hustle John Paul and I found ways to incorporate John's busy life with ours. Often Saturdays and Sundays armed with a picnic basket we joined him at Long Beach, or San Pedro, wherever he happened to be working. My son and I dressed in shorts, tank tops, and bathing suits beneath, ready for a swim in the ocean, and my husband covered in black oil came to meet us on his lunch break or at a change of shifts; the sites had easy access to the beach.

Time zoomed by, and a year and half later John graduated with exceptionally good marks as a petroleum engineer. In a special ceremony with my husband, Alice, and John Paul present, as well as other spouses, I received a P.H.T. (Putting Hubby Through) diploma offered by the University to wives who helped their husbands finish the course.

Scouts from Tide Water Oil Company from Ventura, California, on the lookout for good prospects to hire, put an attractive job offer in front of him. He was put in charge together with other engineers in the firm of looking after the wells in the extended oil fields of Oxnard and Ventura. The toil of the past two years vanished, but the new opportunity implied relocating again.

Eager and happy but at the same time with some sadness, the moment to say good-bye to the two most significant persons involved in my life while in Los Angeles had come: Dr. Dunbar and my dear friend Alice. I promised to stay in touch with them; after all Ventura was only a little over an hour drive away, which I did, I kept my promise.

July, 1985

In the later part of July, John Paul left for France. I expected to have some news from him soon and a little later from Judith. Yet it was difficult to forecast what her answer might be.

Impatiently, the voice that lately had become my regular adviser, rambled, "Time is of essence for you. Who knows if Judith will even accept your business plan; it's unwise to stay immobile!" I knew the murmur was right. I could not just sit and wait for her answer, besides John Paul could call any time requesting the money for the treatment.

"You can get 18 dollars per gram in Brazil," Bernard had said, and it was a tempting quote. So impetuously I resolved to venture a trip to Brazil and explore that option. If anything, it would help me gain some money as well as experience. This was not just a game I was playing; I was coldblooded plotting my incursion into the drug trade, letting the dread of losing my son overrun my principles.

From the moment I reconnected with Jim and met his associates, I kept in touch. I asked questions; they in turn supplied me with information in all areas of the trade, but nothing concrete had come up until now.

Still with some access to American dollars on my credit line, I called Bernard with more specific questions. "I would like to coordinate a meeting with your friend in Brazil. How soon do you think this can happen?" I asked urgently. "I can call Alfonzo right away and arrange a date at your convenience," Bernard responded, in his usual relaxed manner.

Nervously I fired my next question, "How much time do you need to prepare 300 hundred grams?" Only silence at the other end, then I heard Bernard's reassuring words, "If I have the money today, the cocaine will be ready within a week."

"You will have it. Its eleven hundred dollars you will need, right?" I asked "Yes," he said and with his answer still sounding in my ears, I ran to the bank to get the dollars. Bernard had the money in his hands later the same day.

In exchange, he gave me the good news, "I've contacted Alfonzo in Sao Paolo. He has agreed to wait for my call to confirm your arrival date and time." Quickly I checked my appointment's agenda; seeing that I was free the following weekend and that I could flee from home without trouble, I told him, "You can advise your friend that I'll be there Friday, July 2nd. I don't know the exact time, but I will take the last flight from Cochabamba to Santa Cruz and then to Sao Paolo."

"He will be waiting to hear from you the minute you arrive then," Bernard responded and we both shook hands, sealing the deal.

A week went by and I had not heard anything from my son yet; I figured he was still in the search. As for me it was time to get back to Bernard to pick up the cocaine, together with Alfonzo's phone number in Sao Paolo, whom I was to call from the airport to receive further instruction.

In paying the balance owing, Bernard who happened to notice my nervousness said, "Myriam, you don't have to worry about my friend. Alfonzo is trustworthy and not only that, he owes me tons of favors. Believe me, he will treat you well." I had no specific reason but I trusted Jim and his friends, so Bernard's words gave me a lot of reassurance.

He went as far as to caution me, "You must be extremely careful in the way you handle the cocaine. The drug has a strong scent, and the highly trained police dogs placed in airport terminals can easily detect it. It has to be wrapped and sealed air-tightly; otherwise, you could end up in trouble."

I should have been scared; I was not. My rationale didn't leave room for hypothetical thoughts of danger. My only concern was to cover my two days of absence from Cochabamba. John was on a field trip; I didn't need any excuses for him. Patrick, my younger son, thought I was going to a friend's wedding; Daisy, our maid was left in charge of looking after him.

Friday I boarded the flight to Sao Paolo. Fearless I carried one small carry-on bag and a beautiful floral arrangement. The drugs were enclosed in airtight plastic bags, concealed in the ceramic vase under the flowers; a simple housewife covering!

As I approached the Customs check-in desk in Santa Cruz, my heart stopped beating. A good friend of ours, a passenger in the same flight, saw me. Carlos with his usual great smile came over to greet me. Of course he could not help but notice the flower arrangement; moreover he offered to carry it. Speaking with his usual loud voice, laughing said, "Myriam, what do we have here, a ton of cocaine perhaps? Please let me help you!"

Carlos was joking of course, not realizing how close to the truth he was. Horrified, I felt faint as he snatched the arrangement from my hands. I had no chance to refuse his solicitous help. Besides, I would have attracted unwanted attention. He went through customs with my package. I closed my eyes. "Come on Myriam hurry up. Let's board the plane," Carlos said, as usual exuding joy for life. My heart went back in place. I nodded and smiled back with relief. I didn't need to be concerned anymore; the flowers with the cocaine were place inside the plane's fridge.

Throughout the flight Carlos and I exchanged a friendly conversation and we parted ways when we landed in Sao Paolo. My carry-on luggage and the flowers in my hands now went through Immigration and Customs without a problem.

Once my friend was out sight, I found a telephone booth and called Alfonzo. He gave me directions. "Myriam, take a taxi to the Regency Hotel. I have booked a room in your name there. I'll come later to pick up the parcel."

Following Bernard's friend instructions, I lodged at the Regency Hotel. The wait was not long. Alfonzo came and without hardly any small talk, perhaps because I was endorsed by Bernard, he quickly tested and weighed the cocaine; satisfied with the product, he paid in American dollars and left. If a flight had been available, the same night I would have returned home.

Since there wasn't, I stayed overnight counting my blessings. I had done it. I was amazed by the simplicity of the operation and returned triumphantly, reassured that I was dealing with honest people. The Brazilian business transaction left me with a good profit. It allowed me to pay back my credit line, John Paul's airline tickets to France and my trip to Brazil, purchased also on credit; I even had some change left in my hands.

Encouraged by the success of this exchange, I was sure that it would not be long before I had the money needed for John Paul's treatment. But I realized I had to devise a better plan. It would otherwise be too evident if I made continuous trips of this nature to the neighboring country. It could stir up Customs' suspicion, not to mention the time it would take; and time was something else I didn't have.

Carefully I considered all the aspects and in the end I thought best to wait for Judith's response; if her answer was affirmative, the cocaine would go to France, if negative it would go to Spain, where Bernard had other friends. Prices had to be similar, so to reach my monetary goal, one or two trips would be all I needed to make, instead of several if I went to Brazil.

I waited a few more days before I called Judith. Anticipating that this would give John Paul enough time to complete his inquires, even allowing him to go through some examinations and subsequently traveled south, or at least mail my letter. I made sure J.P. had Judith's address.

The interval seemed long, but it was worth while the wait seeing that I was about to get a definite answer from Judith and perhaps the results from my son's search. On the second ring my surrogated cousin answered, and not beating around the bush she said, "I'm interested and John Paul is here; he delivered your letter."

Caught of guard by Judith's swift answer, I had to tell her, "I hope you checked he is not around to hear our conversation; or anyone else for that matter. You need to be sure," I warned her.

"Of course I have. I'm in my den with closed doors," Judith responded and continued, "I've approached one of my friends. She is a frequent guest at rich people's parties and about our specifics, Lydia said, 'It's an attractive idea. I know just the kind of people, but before we go any further, or I contact anyone, I need more details.'"

Naturally Judith now passed those queries to me, "She wants to know what quantities we are talking about and what is the price you expect to get paid per gram? The sooner my friend knows, the faster she will get the contact ready." Wahoo! My speculations had been right; everything was in high gear now.

In regards to the quantity, I hadn't decided yet. Thirty thousand dollars was still my goal, the amount I expected to create from the proceeds after all debts and expenses were paid. So largely it depended on the price I could obtain, "I'm informed the value in Spain is thirty six American dollars per gram; if I can get the same amount through your friend, great. In any event, I'm open to negotiate if it means a quick sale." Boasting with words and knowledge I didn't have, trying to impress her, I added, "We are talking about 700 grams for a start."

"Okay, I will pass the information on to my friend. The minute I hear from her, I'll call you back." Judith responded and we then exchanged a few more superfluous words, and then I asked her, "Will you please put John Paul on the phone?"

My son's voice brought me comfort, but felt saddened when he said, "I didn't learn much Mom, only general information on the topic." Fearful Judith would overhear our conversation John Paul was not too explicit, he instead said, "We will talk about it another time, okay?"

Changing the subject J.P. continued, "If it's okay with you Mom, I would like to stay in Cannes for a while longer. Judith has a few tours on her agenda. I'm already in France, and she is willing to teach me her line of work. Imagine, I could go to Monaco, Rome, and cities in Southern France. I'll learn about the history and the art for which France is so well known and it won't cost me a nickel. I'll be paid instead! It'll be only for a couple weeks?"

John Paul was excited. It was impossible not to notice the new enthusiasm in his voice; I could not refuse his request. "Of course you can stay, dear," I said and after wishing him well we both hung up. I had no problem accepting John Paul's petition, it would at least give him some joy, something else to entertain his thoughts other than his predicament.

The trip had handed out the unexpected; my son felt alive again. He no longer resembled the walking corpse before mentioned, with no desire for anything from life. Even if my son's queries had not been overly successful, it gave me hope. Besides and regardless of my dire financial situation I had already taken the resolution, the quest in France had to evolve; it would be only a matter of time before I succeeded. John Paul's condition had to be treated no matter what."

January, 1965

THE HOUSE WITH THE WHITE PICKET FENCE CAME ALONG WITH the relocation. A small down payment helped us purchase a three-bedroom rancher in a new subdivision; children playing around in the front yards prompted us in favor of this place. John Paul, who at the nursery had mastered the art of socializing, couldn't be more thrilled. The minute we moved into the house, we had kids from next door and from across the street move into our backyard!

John and I were also excited; the Californians' affability matched by our own opened many doors. Soon we had good friends and to put the icing on the cake, my relationship with my husband blossomed. We loved each other, but the rapport we had for one another went well beyond; we found pleasure in being in each other's company as good friends do.

I suppose we had the right ingredients; for one, we were young, happy and always eager to do more. John's work was now Monday through Friday and most every evening he was also at home. Stimulated by my husband's enthusiasm for adventures, on weekends I was just as keyed up as John Paul to head out on excursions. California had a vast territory to explore and while John studied we didn't do much; it was catching up time.

Malibu beach was one of our favorite hang-outs, as well as Santa Barbara, a city I love for its Spanish flare and where I felt almost at home. Or we went towards the mountains, where our hikes took us to astoundingly views. I was satisfied.

At Christmas, we never failed to visit John's parents, we only needed to gas-up the car and go; even after our first frightening experience as we almost froze to death in the Californian car we traveled. The one we bought as a second car when in L.A. was comfortable but had no winter insulation; therefore along the way to the **North Pole,** it turned into a deepfreeze. But no matter, the 30 hours drive to Calgary was well worth it. Family ties were fortified and our son experienced at least the love of one set of grandparents. In addition John's stepdad, fixed up our car so that it was on par for both Californian and Canadian weather.

To visit my parents was not that simple; travel that far was on the expensive side, more so multiplied by three. My connection with them, my sister and friends, was through the old snail way, letters, given that long distance calls to South America were still in the air. Often the operator would say, "Your call is through now," only to hear unnervingly static noises coming from the phone.

I was definitely lonely for physical contact with my family; my cousin Raul's presence broke somewhat this isolation. He had immigrated to the States earlier on, residing in San Bernardino with his wife and his five children. At first I was not too eager to reconnect with him; in our adolescence my sister and I bumped heads with him. Older than us, too serious and rigid with his principles, Raul constantly was on our case; apparently our *attributes* were not of his liking. However my nostalgia won over; I put those stupid quarrels from the past aside and decided to look him up.

What a grand get-together we had then with him, his wife Lila and their growing family. John had only met Raul in L.A, but their engineering backgrounds bonded them immediately. As frequently as my husband's studies permitted we went to see them. Loretta their youngest and John Paul of almost the same age got along splendidly. Now in Ventura we saw them more often, the visits went each way but our reconnection was short lived. Raul and his family decided to go back to Bolivia.

Once again I found work. The excellent references Dr. Dunbar, my previous boss, gave me helped a lot. My husband had no objections this time; John Paul's kindergarten time and my work schedule didn't conflict

Hired as a medical assistant by Dr. J. Walker a heart specialist, and Dr. M, Phillips, a psychiatrist, both shared the premises and I shared the workload with Jean Martin, the RN, who in no time became a close friend. More and more I adapted to the life in Ventura and it soon began to feel like home.

John and Walter, Jean's husband, inevitably met, and a strong camaraderie grew between them. Our new friends had five children; J.P. was still our only one and loved to be around them. They happened to go to the same school, John Paul and Leslie the youngest of the bunch even attended the same class and became inseparable.

With hardly any planning, we ended up getting together on the weekends. BBQs happened at the spur of the moment at our home or theirs; some weekends we even went camping together. My husband's stories mainly about his experiences in Bolivia, where he saw the great importance people gave to family values, plus the enjoyment he'd found in my country, pepped up the gatherings and kept his audience in awe.

Walter, a carpenter by trade but a farmer by heart, quizzically but attentively listened to my husband's exposés and intrigued inquired, "Tell me John, what kind of opportunity does a person like me would have in Bolivia?" "Unlimited! You should see the vast amounts of fantastic farm and ranch land available at very low cost. People in Bolivia, with enough know how, hard work, and tools can easily become rich in a short time. The possibilities for lucrative businesses are countless," my husband responded with a dreamy look on his face.

John could expound on the subject for hours and no one was bored. The topic drew a lot of interest; our friends wanted to know more, especially Walter, who always came up with more questions. Jean joined in the quiz a bit later and then both were mesmerized by John's anecdotes. He spoke so highly of my country that I even got to fantasizing!

In no time the realm of dreams changed and degrees, diplomas, all of John's latest accomplishment would end on the back burner for now. From what I already knew of my husband, his new vision had to do more with a dream he had in his youth: to have a cattle ranch! The foresight became contagious; one thing led to another and as time went by, the Martins and we seriously began to consider relocating our families to a new life in Bolivia.

There was not much we could do from where we stood; for starters we needed fresh information. The how and where to enquire was a bit complex. Telephone communication between the north and the looked down-on southern relatives continued to be a trial. The only other resort was the well-known route, the snail mail way.

In a long letter father got entrusted with the investigation: find land prices in the Santa Cruz vicinity as soon as possible. The plan was to establish a self-sufficient cattle ranch that would support both our families and provide employment to locals.

Dad's response letter brought us astonishing news. The Bolivian government was working on an experimental project that seemed to fit like a glove with our own. To attract foreign investment in the country, mainly in agriculture, they were opening undeveloped areas; their aim was to create a steady source of income for local peasants. The regulations for prospective investors were simple; the enterprise had to be incorporated as a local legal entity in order to receive the free land and tax cuts.

The dream became an idea and now an incredible reality, something beyond our expectations. The land wouldn't cost us a nickel! Our good friends the Martins and ourselves, eager to do something more with our lives, had now the opportunity to change the story and attain the unattainable: build a castle in the sky!

Elated, we could not believe our luck. What's more is that the Bolivian president, a colonel in the air force happened to be a friend of my family and having paid attention to my father's enquires told him, "If Myriam, her husband and her group are genuinely interested, I will personally oversee their endeavor and ensure all possible assistance. Keep me informed, Guillermo."

Immediately we and the Martins had a lawyer draw up the corporate papers. The documents, including the study of our own project prepared by professionals in the field, and our plan for our future investments, plus the power of attorney for my father to represent us, were in governmental hands now. Dad personally had delivered the portfolio.

By return mail the Ministry of Agriculture, through my father, informed us that our project had been accepted and that we have been granted fifty thousand hectares! The ministerial people were talking about hectares, not acres. It would take a lifetime for anyone to put that much land to use. It was likely just a mistake, so our response went in a short missive, "We thank you for considering and accepting our project, however we are under the impression the grant is far too excessive; ten thousand hectares should be more than enough to complete our goal."

The officer in charge, who seemed to know more about our needs than us, recommended, "Your enterprise should at least have twenty thousand hectares; we will draw the papers for this amount. The closing document would be finalized with your own signatures upon your arrival." If they wanted to be that generous, it was fine with us. We didn't contradict his authority any longer and accepted the Ministerial offer.

It was a tremendous amount of land and nothing less than in the best ranching land. John happened to have worked in the area in 1958; apparently scattered tall flowering hardwood trees and some lower brush broke the wild grass pastures. The grant had about 20 kilometers along the **Rio Grande**, eight kilometers of railroad frontage, and a patch of terrain that could easily be cleared for a landing strip. We had hit the jackpot, but then again surely the government realized the benefit our venture would bring to the people in the surrounding areas.

Ignited by the good news, Walter and John worked like dynamos. In any spare time they went to auctions looking for deals; they bought a six-ton truck, a caterpillar tractor, a large generator, welding equipment, two water pumps, plus other machinery and tools, all purchased at exceptionally good prices.

Attracted by our efforts, the two doctors Jean and I worked for got involved, and together with other friends in the field donated medical equipment and supplies for our project. Since our goal was to be self sufficient, Jean felt confident we could start a small walk-in clinic; the idea would benefit mostly the people living nearby. Presently no one had any access to this kind of service.

At first only the Martins and us were engaged in the project, but soon another couple joined in; Mike and Michelle who had two small children. They were interested in the traveling part of the adventure, not in settling in Bolivia. Soon Terry, my husband's cousin from Alberta and his friend Tom, jumped on board saying, "Will you please take us along, we wouldn't want to miss an adventure such as this." Terry had heard of our expedition through John's mother

The green light from my father came in the later part of July. The Ministry of Agriculture had completed the paperwork for the grant. It had taken 16 months and now our presence in Bolivia was needed to sign the final documents.

We vacated our previously sold homes and we were now ready to journey the thousands of kilometers to Panama. The plan was to continue the rest of the voyage on an ocean liner, aiming for a port in Peru with access to local roads given that our final destination was Bolivia.

A few days before our departure, reporters from local newspapers aware of our exciting adventure visited us and took pictures of all 15 members of the expedition, including the six hardy vehicles...and in the flash of a camera we became celebrities!

AUGUST, 1985

ON AUGUST 10, JOHN PAUL CAME BACK FROM FRANCE EXHAUSTED. The trip had been very long, but before heading to his room to rest, J.P. relayed to his father, Patrick, and I, some of the great experiences he'd had with Judith, thanks to her line of work. He then crashed 'til the next day.

The next morning, after John had left for work and Patrick to school, I went to John Paul's room and in private, I listened to the details on the real reason for his trip, "As planned Mom, I visited the Louis Pasteur Institute but it was fruitless; they don't just accept anyone that walks in the door without some kind of referral." From the frown on my son's forehead, I gathered the difficulties he must have experienced.

He took a deep breath, and as he spoke again J. P.'s face got somber. "Soon I found that France, much the same as the United States, has higher medical costs for non-residents, and as you well know Mom, I didn't have that sort of money, the kind that opens all doors. Despite this fact, I brought back some literature on the AIDS research from the Pasteur Institute." His thoughts wandered off again, while I quietly waited not quite realizing yet what he had gone through.

"It's not easy to try and locate a doctor not speaking the language, besides risking rejection. I experienced that too Mom." I could hardly hear my son speak now, so I moved closer to him as he muttered the next words, "You should have seen the reaction of a receptionist, when I told her I needed to see the doctor for a referral for the Pasteur Institute, because I thought I had AIDS! She just pointed me to the door. After that I had no courage and left. I didn't pursue any further. Instead I went directly to visit Judith in Cannes and I'm happy I did."

Though all had been so intense, I noticed John Paul seemed untroubled, as if the lack of a positive result in France didn't affect him. It was as though his illness had passed to a second level. In closing he said, "Mom I don't want to speak about it any more."

John Paul then with a placid smile on his face asked me to go back in time. "Mom, do you remember when I was only a little boy and Dad was at the wheel of the car driving through the oil fields in Alberta; you and I sat next to him as happy passengers listening to the radio, while Doris Day softly sang,

"When I was just a little boy, I asked my father, what would I be? Would I be rich, would I be poor, and he said could be? *Que sera, sera...* whatever will be, will be, the future is not ours to see, what will be will be..."

"It could be Mom that this illness will be the cause of my death. It might also be that scientists guided by God, will soon discover the cure; then all our worries will be over. In any event, we need to keep on living. Okay! Do you understand, Mom? We don't know what the future will hold for us, right? But I do know that it won't be as bad, if you promise to stop worrying about me. I can't bear the thought that I'm the cause of your suffering. Shall we try to put my illness behind us and enjoy life, one day at a time?"

I was deeply moved by my son's speech and oh, how I wished I could make John Paulito be better again as I used to do when he was that little boy and I soothed his bruises with the magic of my love. But it was different now.

After those words he kissed me and went back to his room while I went to work. But I had no intentions in abandoning the hunt! The articles about Rock Hudson's condition never stated that he did not find the cure. It was imperative then that I obtain the funds to continue on with my search. Everything was possible with money! My son's monologue dug deep in my heart, it hurt, but it gave me a new revitalizing energy.

I still had tried to obtain the money lawfully, by approaching a couple of bank managers for a credit line, good friends, who many times in the past had granted John and I the credit backed-up only by a written agreement. But naturally now my request was denied, the country's economy was chaotic and bankers didn't want to take any risks.

To sell some assets was not a possibility, not only for lack of buyers but also because the properties were in partnership with Mauricio. Out of the question, it would mean a lot of explaining to give and necessarily the truth about my son would come out.

Judith's intended visit to her father was in mid-September. "Just be patient for a little longer," I told myself attempting to calm my nerves, trusting her friend by then would have a buyer for the cocaine, but the mañana, mañana didn't seem to come fast enough for me.

The buzzing of a phone ringing interrupted my present ongoing routine, endlessly thinking. "Oh. Hi Judith," I said, hoping my heart would stop beating so loud with the anticipation of her response. "I will be in La Paz next Tuesday. I'll stay with my Father for over a week and I'll come over to see you after. I need to place my order for the crafts now. Do you have a pen handy?" I could care less about her order, what I wanted was to hear was the other stuff, but containing my impatience I answered, "Yes I do, shoot."

Done with her order, Judith jovially told me, "My friend has found someone who is interested. She wants to be only a go between and be paid for her troubles. The customer is willing to pay up to thirty American dollars per gram, but no more. About the quantity, it is up to you, but I mentioned it would probably be 700 grams to start. It's what you told me right? Whatever the amount it'll be fine with them; my friend will be happy to arrange the deals." I digested Judith's words and eager for immediate results, I decided I would accept their price, but I was not sure about the quantity, or how and by who the drug would be transported and delivered.

It didn't take long before the *guru* I now had within me to whisper a hint, "Why don't you ask Judith to do it?" A brilliant idea! It would not only save me the airfare, but also the explanations if it were me who had to travel. But again it was a tricky subject to discuss with Judith over the phone; it was best if I waited for her arrival. Besides it would be easier to check her reaction. In any event if her response was negative, I had no qualms about taking the drug myself.

"Great Judith, I will have your order ready and we will talk about the other stuff too. Will talk about the whole thing when you get here. See you then." My friend's report was all I needed to set myself in motion.

The three hundred grams I took to Brazil proved to be a small package; the 700 hundred mentioned didn't seem a lot more, volume wise. Likely the right amount, still safe and profitable.

Lacking the credit from the banks, beforehand I had investigated other source, a person who loaned money in American currency. Since now things were coming into place, I visited him. Introductions aside I asked, "Victor, I need ten thousand dollars." His ugly face became alive the minute I mention my need and his cavernous smile grew as he answered back, "No problem Mrs. Arthur but you should know that the interest I charge is ten per cent per month. Are you still interested?"

I am not sure what impacted me the most, that hideous smile or the excessively high interest rate. I wished I did not need to deal with this loan shark, but with my back against a wall, I did not see any other way to secure the money. "Yes I am. What do I have to do?" I asked him.

"For security purposes, you will sign a promissory note and bring some of your jewelry. It will serve as collateral." Victor licked his lips as if already testing the catch, he actually had a big mouth and now his gigantic smile gave to his oral cavity the look of a true shark, scary!

The next day I brought a few pieces of my jewelry, indeed more in value than the ten thousand dollars I received in the exchange. I had no second thoughts about leaving my treasures with him. I could not just sell the jewels myself; after all they were presents from John, he would ask questions if they vanished. Besides I was confident my jewels would be back in place once my transaction in France was completed and I reimbursed Victor. So I closed the deal.

Cash in hand I immediately set off to see my suppliers, "Jim, I brought the money for the 700 grams' initial payment, my friend requested; as I told you over the phone he wants his identity concealed. I'm here on his behalf. I'll bring the balance in a week's time. You will have the cocaine ready then, right?" In order to protect my steps, I had come up with that story. Jim nodded, while he counted the money.

As if nothing troubled me, I continued to work and maintained a stable household. After school Patrick would bring a bunch of his friends home; the big yard around the house was appropriate for all types of games and our home was filled with laughter. Whereas John Paul, immersed in his drawings and paintings was oblivious of my plan. I had not told him anything, so J.P. had no idea that once I had the money he was returning to France. Thankfully his health seemed to indicate that he was still doing fine.

Some of my **good** friends, because of my son's prolonged stay in Bolivia, began to ask questions. "Isn't John Paul returning to California?" one busy body inquired, while another in a sarcastic tone just as aggravating snooped, "Is John Paul now staying for good in Cochabamba? Didn't you mention he had an interesting job in Hollywood?"

Irritated by their prying, I vigorously responded, "No, he is not staying. Soon he will return to California and resume his work as a makeup artist for Universal Studios, and will also continue with his studies. He wants to major in Special Effects; his goal is to become a director like Spielberg, but right now John Paul is having a well-deserved vacation." After my response, the ladies didn't enquire any more; I suppose because their questions backfired.

That would have been J. P.'s plan before, but not now. My so call friends' curiosity had given me a hard reality check. Until then, I had not given a thought to the time ahead. For the moment my only concern was the present, to have my son well again. The rest was in limbo.

On september 11, Judith arrived. My family and I were happy to see her again. She updated us with news on her loved ones, "Jean Christian is now eight and Olivia four. I left them in Cannes. My mother in-law is staying in my house looking after them."

"Where is your husband now?" I asked. "Jean Pierre is still in Africa, I believe in Nigeria, where he has been working for the past three months. He hopes to return to France and rejoin us for Christmas but nothing's certain yet." After the chitchat, Judith and I were left alone to discuss business in private.

"Tell me about your friend," I asked, starting to fire off innumerable questions. "From where do you know her? Does she understand everything well?" Judith calmly and in few words filled in the gaps for me. "I met my friend at a party. We both frequented parties of well-to-do people. After the day's tour, my routine is to take rich American travelers to the homes of these people, with whom the agency has made arrangements. It as a way to give the tourists a taste of French lifestyle; this woman was part of the crowd and we became friends."

"One more question Judith," I prodded. Do you know your friend well, enough to trust her? Remember, we have to be extremely careful with the stuff we deal." "Oh don't worry Myriam my friend is trustworthy. If I approached her, it is because I knew she needed money. Her pay-out demand for connecting you with people in the business will be a ten percent of the total sale."

It all sounded reasonable and Judith's responses totally satisfied me I was convinced that Judith got the right person, dependable and trustworthy. For some unknown reason I felt safer dealing with a person like her, a woman from high society, rather than with Bernard's contact!

With that settled I put in front of my friend my next plan of attack, except that Judith didn't want anything to do with transporting and delivering the cocaine. In fact, she outright refused. "Are you crazy Myriam? I certainly won't do it. I could be caught!" she said in a high-pitched voice.

I'd sort of expected her response. Such a suggestion would have scared anyone, but with a bit of persuasion I was sure I could make her change her mind and overcome the fear. "Judith, there is nothing to worry about. I've done it myself not too long ago; I went to Sao Paolo with three hundred grams." Concentrating on the savings her help would represent, I pushed a little further. I went so far as to explain in detail my experience.

She still refused, but seemed curious. Seeing that I might still be able to convince her, I continued, "I assure you, I don't foresee any problems as long as you confide only in the people referred to you by your friend." It was natural for me to be so confident. I was on my own crusade, therefore my mission was both logical and foolproof and for the same reason I didn't consider myself a drug dealer.

My intention was to supply the cocaine to people in high society, who in my knowledge only used it socially. I drilled this position into Judith's head strongly, but it was only after I had showed her the way I had camouflaged the cocaine that she finally accepted.

Once I picked up the 700 grams of cocaine, I took Bernard's advice literally, "No scent should escape from the packaging," he'd said, but didn't suggest how I should to do it. Inspired as ever I got a bottle of hair shampoo and another of hair conditioner. First I poured out the substances inside, then in succession carefully installed three 10cm x 20cm plastic bags; one bag inside the other in the now vacant vessels, making sure the open ends remained at the mouth of the bottles.

Using a tiny spoon I patiently filled the cocaine into the interior of the last bag placed. When it felt well packed, I sealed it, then sealed the next, and the next, one after the other. Carefully, to ensure that neither shampoo nor conditioner would seep into the plastic bags, since any space left in between, I refilled it with the original matter.

If anyone happened to open the containers they would only find shampoo and conditioner and be unaware that one bottle held four hundred grams of cocaine and the other three hundred. How did I manage to concoct such deceptive covering on my own? I don't have a clue! My newly-acquired creativity surmounted my own expectations. It looked perfect.

To prove my point I asked Judith "Do you see anything suspicious in these bottles?" "No, I don't," she answered with a puzzled look on her face. It was then that I explained what it contained and what exactly I had done with them, and Judith raised her eyebrows in disbelief.

Not only I had to convince her that it was safe to transport it. It was also important Judith knew the packaging aspect in detail, so that once in France she would know how to retrieve the drug. It had to be carefully done. Otherwise the bags could break and the cocaine would be damaged. I had to prevent such an accident and loss; it would jeopardize the whole purpose of my plan.

Still undecided Judith had some questions of her own. "What will happen if the police in France, or in any of the countries I have to go through, detect the white powder? What would I do then?"

"I don't anticipate anything going wrong, but if by any circumstances it's detected and you are questioned, you have to maintain ignorance. You would only say, "I delegated the purchase and the packaging of the crafts to someone in Bolivia. I'm not aware of any other packages," I responded with confidence.

Nevertheless I certainly didn't want her to do anything unless it was of her own free will. "If you still think this is too risky, you don't have to go along with any of it. You can just drop the whole thing right now. I can take care of it myself. Yet, if you decide to take part, it is better you understand that there are some risks involved," I said looking straight into her eyes.

Everything sounded so simple, no wonder Judith after a few more minutes was all for my idea. We then proceeded to discuss the percentage of her profit and our conversation ended with a fair agreement for both of us.

When Judith and I joined the rest of the family we discovered some friends had dropped by and were gathered in a cheerful conversation. I am not sure if my next words came out as preventive measure, or to maintain the status we had, but instinctively I announced, "Judith and I have decided to be partners in an export business venture. We plan to introduce some Bolivian artisan's work to France."

"That is wonderful Myriam, we wish you great success." The group gleefully supported us. More and more I was becoming a queen in the art of deceit. A few days later Judith left for France with the artisan crafts and the cocaine.

AUGUST, 1966

JOHN, DRIVING OUR FOUR-WHEEL F-350 PICKUP TRUCK WITH A self contained camper was at the head of the convoy. John Paul was not yet six and I sat next to him; Mike and Michelle and their two children followed behind us in their Land Rover.

Jean was driving their F-350, which the same as ours had their living accommodation on board. Leslie and Marlene, the youngest and the second youngest daughters with her. Terry drove the F-150 pickup truck with a smaller camper on top; accompanying him, Teresa the oldest Martin girl. Tom his friend, drove the other Land Rover: with him the older Martin boy. Walter completed the caravan driving the Ford-600 truck; carrying boxed-in at the back all the tools and small equipment not shipped to Bolivia by freight cargo. With him traveled his two younger sons.

Our aim was to get to Bolivia as quickly as possible, thus we had no intention to explore Aztec sights or search for Spanish traditional towns. Switching drivers every so often and having only a few overnight stopovers was the plan to swiftly leave behind the thousands of kilometers separating us from our final destination.

Mexico was the start of our itinerary, then Guatemala, El Salvador, Honduras, Nicaragua, Costa Rica, and Panama. To expedite border crossing for our caravan, the Minister of External Affairs in Bolivia sent letters to the Ministerial counterparts in all of these countries, requesting free-passage through their territory for our equipment, luggage, and vehicles; my father made sure we had copies of the dispatch in our hands.

As we crossed into Tijuana, our point of entry into the Aztec territory, the obstacles began. Immigration and Customs officials, speaking only Spanish, requested documents and papers for the vehicles. Except for John and I, the rest of our party didn't have an idea as to what was being said. It was then that with no other alternative on hand that instantly I became the official interpreter for the group.

The officer in charge recognized having received a letter from the higher-ups in Mexico City acknowledging the free passage for our caravan, but seemingly not in the expected fashion. In Spanish he blabbered, "Your convoy can go through Mexico but only if it's escorted by a Custom Official." He then added that the favor didn't come free, "You will need to pay the officer twenty dollars per day, supply him with food, and pay his way back."

It took me a while to integrate all he said and then translate the unexpected news to John and our partners. Their mouths dropped open in disbelief; the not budgeted expense didn't sit well with any of us, nor the idea of having a stranger mingled with us in close quarters during the duration of the trip through Mexico.

We had no other choice than to accept the mandate. But John who had already found a solution to minimized the problem said, "To cut down on the expense, we just have to put pedal to the metal and speed through Mexico." He then looking at a map added, "It took us four hours to drive the six hundred kilometers plus from Ventura to Tijuana; we should stop and rest only every 1400 kilometers. So the town of Caborca will be our next stop; then Culiacan, followed by Guadalajara, and Puebla will be our last. This way we will be at the Guatemalan border in five days.

As scheduled by the third day, speeding moderately, we got to Guadalajara. It was a beautiful colonial Spanish style city, though the narrow streets highly predominant in the downtown core didn't handle heavy traffic well. We studied the road maps beforehand, but inadvertently we had entered into this zone and our convoy got cut off while crossing a busy intersection; three vehicles went through on the green light, but the other three were left behind.

Not too concerned, the now divided convoy continued forward. We had a two-way radio system, the latest transmitting device, specifically installed in all vehicles to keep the group connected while on route. Above and beyond every driver knew that our next destination was the city of Toluca, a few miles before Mexico City. This was a vital stop as any mail was to be delivered to the town's main post office.

We just had to look for road signs pointing to Toluca and followed them. "Beep, Beep," the two-way radio sounded, "Myriam, can you hear me? We are now crossing the last intersection and we can't see you. How far behind are you anyway?" John didn't wait to hear my response, he just rattled on.

"We won't wait for you; there is too much traffic. We'll just meet before entering the highway to Toluca. See you there." My husband's voice came loud and clear, our son was with him. Jean and her girls as well as Mike and his family were in that group of vehicles. "Okay," I responded. I was with Walter in the big truck and the rest of the boys in the other two vehicles; drivers as well as passengers we all rotated.

Walter looked at me and we both smiled, silently understanding that he had to push harder on the gas pedal to catch up with them. The city limit behind us now, and going down a hill nothing obstructed our view, yet there was no sign of the frontward group. Suddenly the truck swirled from one side of the road to the other; dangerously leaning on the driver's side, ready to roll over. Walter somehow managed to control the vehicle and was able to stop it before it happened.

All shook-up we got out, followed by the other guys from the other vehicles. We looked for the damage and found that the truck had lost its back left dual wheels and in doing so broke the axle. But luck had been on our side; had the truck rolled over, it would have been fatal. Walter an expert driver had steered clear and the incident ended just as a mechanical accident.

The other group had to be informed. Beep, beep, I sounded the radio, but only static noises came through the waves. I tried again and again, no response. Walter, Terry, and Tom, huffing and puffing, put in place the hoist at the front of the pickup truck and with the help of the winch the axle was successfully removed.

Except for the two-way radio device that ceased to function, we had good tools; but right now we had no means to notify our problem to the rest of the caravan and that we were heading back into Guadalajara to have the axle repaired. The truck, jacked up and secured, was left at the side of the road with a note for John, explaining everything and telling him we would connect at the trailer park where we'd stayed the previous night. Naturally we figured that once they realized we were not coming they would retrace their steps, then find the truck and the note.

The trailer park facility was a point of reference, so naturally as soon as we got back to town, it was our first stop. I rang the bell at the caretaker's unit and explained, "We had a mechanical setback right after we left this morning; our vehicle is being repaired now. Has anyone been looking for us?" I asked, "No. No one has been here," the attendant responded and I spoke again. "When the rest of our group calls, or comes looking for us, will you tell them what happened to us and that we are parked in the outskirts of town on the road heading for Toluca. We have set up camp there." He agreed to do so.

For the next three days while the axle was being fixed, we made sure to check with the clerk and each time he just shook his head and said, "Sorry, no, they haven't come or called, but if they do I'll certainly pass the message."

Walter scratched his head and said, "Well if they haven't shown up they probably thought we drove directly to Toluca; by now likely they are waiting for us there." Concerned but maintaining optimism I responded, "Yes, we'll just have to wait until then and check at the post office. I'm sure we'll find a note telling us where they are." With no other way to contact the rest of our party and as a precaution, we left a message at the police station in case John attempted to check on us through them.

Once our truck was fixed, we frantically drove to Toluca to regroup with our loved ones, but no one had stopped at the post office. There was no note from them. Not a good sign! Only then did it dawn on me; my husband was not the type to remain silent or inactive while his wife was out of touch. Something terribly wrong must have happened. Immediately, we went to the police station to check with the Mexican police to find out if they knew the whereabouts of our families.

"Oh Lord. Please don't let this be true!" I pleaded with God as the words the police officer sank in. *"Lo siento senora pero tengo que informarle que ha ocurrido un accidente fatal en el camino a Toluca. Una camioneta cayo en el barranco; dos de los ocupantes estan muertos, y dos fueron llevados al hospital."*

I went through shock, disbelief, and panic. I could not accept what I was told. To intensify my distress, everything said was in Spanish and now in agonizing pain I had to repeat the news in English to Walter, his two sons, Terry and Tom, when all I wanted to do was scream and cry but I had to do it. "They just informed me that a fatal accident has occurred on the road to Toluca. A pickup truck went down an embankment, two of the occupants are dead, and two are at the hospital," I ended sobbing.

A police who seemed to have some knowledge of English intervene, "Can I do anything to help?" He said and I managed to ask him; praying that all this was a big mistake and that the news was not really for us. "How do you know those are the people we are looking for?"

"They are *gringos*, traveling in a caravan with other vehicles and the license plates are from California. All this information seems to coincide with the people you are looking for." The officer's dry response was not encouraging. Stressed out, still hoping all was just a big mistake I asked again, "Do you have the names of the dead and the ones wounded?" "I'm sorry; no. You'll have to go back to Guadalajara and find out for yourselves." We left the precinct with those final words still echoing in our ears.

Now we knew the reason for their silence. My whole being was contracted in pain; it could not be that my husband and son were the ones dead, it just could not be! In agony I cursed the moment my husband made the decision to venture on this journey.

No one in the group felt in any condition for the long drive back to Guadalajara, we were too distressed. We decided to take the bus instead. It was late in the afternoon. The streets were abandoned, heavy rain poured down as if the heavens had opened up to flood the earth once again, getting murky by the minute. We stood at the bus stop waiting for one that would take us back to Guadalajara.

In this gloomy stage, out of nowhere three vehicles went by speeding-up through the desert street heading out of town. I rubbed my eyes to clear my vision. Walter did the same and everyone else did too, not sure if what we just saw was real. We could not all be having the same delusion; those vehicles that like phantoms went by were the missing ones from our group.

They were all safe then! Walter, the boys and I laughed and cried with relief and happiness. We yelled, screamed, we jumped up and down raising our arms trying to no avail to attract the drivers' attention, but they continued to drive away.

A taxi happened to cross by, we signaled the driver to stop. Once inside I ordered him in Spanish; now translated to English, "Please follow those vehicles, my husband and son are in one of them." Obeying my orders, he goes in pursuit of the cars, while I explained our entire ordeal. Understanding, he sped through the streets trying to catch up with them; we couldn't lose them again!

The cab driver now quite involved in our pursuit sped some more, going even through red lights. He did not want to lose sight of the vehicles and gained on them. Finally, after continuously honking, he passed them, swirled around and stopped in front of John's vehicle; he was the one at the lead. Luckily there was not much traffic; the torrential rain had kept people indoor otherwise we could have caused a serious accident.

I jumped out of the cab and in seconds I was banging on the pickup's closed window. My husband, who only now realized I was the cause of the chaos, leaped out of the truck and both unconcerned of the rain, soaked to the skin, hugged one another. I could not speak, my heart seemed to have vaulted into my throat and all I could do was sob and laugh.

John was not speaking either; his eyes seemed watery and there was something unusual about his normal confident poise, so I asked, "Why do you have such look of a concern on your face John?"

My husband kept silent and just continued to hold me tightly in his arms. He then clearing his throat said, "We only arrived in town two hours ago and of course we went to the post office looking for some news from you, a note or something letting us know of your whereabouts. There was nothing! It was strange and also unnerving; we had no other way to find you than to go to the police and inquire, only to learn that a serious accident involving your group had occurred some miles out of Guadalajara. Myriam, my God! I thought you were dead."

John Paulito who seemed as if he just woke up, rubbing his eyes crawled out of the vehicle saying, "Mom, Mom you are here!" and the three of us, hugging and kissing, danced under the rain, while the rest of the entire group did the same.

We paid the taxi driver, thanked him for all his help and dispatched him. Once I got into the vehicle with my husband and son, John filled me as to what happened to them. "A few kilometers out of Guadalajara, the Land Rover halted on us; it had to do with the four wheel drive. It forced us to return to the city to have it fixed! When I couldn't get out anything out of the two-way radios, I told Jean "These damn radios, I can't hear a thing. They're probably out of reach, or these things aren't working. I'm sure they'll drive a few more miles and unable to find us they'll turn around to check on what has happened to us."

"We waited three days for the part to arrive and the Rover to be fixed. In that time, either Jean or I went to the trailer park to check for messages from someone from your group, and left ours, telling the attendant, "When the rest of our group calls, or comes looking for us, tell them we had a mechanical problem and that we are parked on the road heading for Toluca." John left this message; same story as ours, but altogether a different situation, an incredible coincidence!

It never dawned on us, nor anyone else to ever mention that there were three different routes heading out from Guadalajara to Toluca; our road maps were not that specific. The realization came only when we all got together again. The accident actually happened and the people involved were Californians vacationing in Mexico

The rest of our travel through Mexico was of a normal nature. It took us twelve days to cross the country instead of the five planned, and except for the time in Guadalajara, where we saw fragments of the city and later the picturesque Santa Vera Cruz, we didn't do a whole lot in Mexico apart from zooming by with the Customs agent as our chaperon whom we bade farewell to at the Guatemalan border.

It was smooth sailing through Central America, other than for a couple of favorable enhancements; the letter for free passage worked wonders in San Salvador. Apparently the country was compromised with political unrest, intense rioting happening everywhere, so no sooner did we presented our documents, emigration officers obeying orders from the Salvadorian government arranged for motorized police escort for our protection, and at no cost to us. Consequently our caravan passed through their territory well protected, which made us feel very important.

In Costa Rica the reception had another stimulating feature: a wealthy landlord, who somehow learned of our plans for ranching in Bolivia, invited us to visit his cattle ranch. He must have seen the potential of our group, because he came up with the idea that we should stay in Costa Rica instead. "Our government can help you achieve your objectives here quicker than in Bolivia, where I understand everything still could be uncertain." He said while he unfolded some maps, "You can find good land over all this area: ranching and cattle land, like mine."

The rancher continued showing us different areas on the map, adding, "I'm sure you can obtain just as good governmental assistance here." All very tempting, however our project was in Bolivia and we were not about to change our minds. Appreciatively we thanked him for his offer and continued forward to Panama.

Because of the uncertainty of our arrival date in Panama, we had not booked in advance tickets or transportation for our vehicles on an ocean liner. Again it turned out that our good fortune was on our side. An Italian transatlantic liner seemed to be waiting for us: first stop Buenaventura in Colombia, and the second the port of Callao in Lima, our destination. The *Milano,* was mainly a cargo ship, but also had passenger accommodations, exactly what we needed!

We boarded the liner, vehicles included. The voyage came with the experience of navigating through the *Panama Canal,* impressive as well as very rewarding considering what came after, at least for me: five miserable wretched days. From day one, the rocking of the boat got me tremendously seasick. I found some solace if I remained lying horizontally in my cot, reading, but the confinement in the small cabin bellow water level, was not pleasant either, it flared up my claustrophobic sense.

For my husband and the rest it was a complete different story, they all had a great time, including John Paul, who when he was not tended to by his father, was always well looked after by someone else in the group.

Moreover when the ship docked in Buenaventura, apparently the two older Martins kids witnessed a smuggling scheme. They saw some nautical people pulled baskets from a small motorboat stationed at one side of the ship, containing what appeared to be whisky bottles, and in return lowered small plastic bags filled with money to pay for the exchange.

Taking advantage of an existing confusion, the boys mischievously robbed from the robbers a couple of bottles, and immediately handed them over to Walter, John, and Mike who sat together enjoying the late morning breeze. They certainly didn't bother to return the loot, instead not wasting any time engulfed the liquid element and had a party, rocking the boat on their own!

I survived their celebration, as well as those endless days, reading a bit and thinking on the treat I knew waited for me in Lima: to see my sister and her family, who lived in *Miraflores*, a suburban district in Lima one hour or so away from Callao, the port where the Milano will dock and our troop disembark.

The plan was to have a restful time with them while provisions were made with railway cargo to have the equipment previously shipped from California (stationed now at the Peruvian yard) to be transported to Bolivia.

In a telegram dispatched from the liner, we informed Vicky and Raul the date and approximate time of our arrival, they were aware of our project. As a result both waited for at the dock and welcomed us with open arms. John, John Paul, and I stayed at their house, while the rest of our comrades and vehicles set up camp on the grounds of a manufacturing plant owned by one of their friends.

They couldn't be more happy to see us, but my sister and Raul were also concerned. My brother in-law pressed by what he thought was irresponsible behavior forthright told us, "You must be out of your minds to embark on such a venture." Realizing he had been a bit too harsh, changing his tone and somewhat laughing added, "Or is it that you have gypsy blood running through your veins?"

Then again in a more serious note he continued, "John, you have continually moved your family from one place to another. Understandable because of your work and studies, but now going ranching, abandoning everything you accomplished before and to go where? To the middle of nowhere?" He spoke in disbelief looking to my sister for support; who just nodded agreeing with him.

I quietly chuckled thinking *and they haven't yet even heard our adventure in Mexico!* Some of my sister's friends, who shared their views, often warmly called us gypsies too. After all who wouldn't? Our caravan consisted of fifteen people and if you added the six vehicles, they all had a good reason to consider us a band of *gitanos*.

Neither John nor I were offended, nor felt rebuked by them. We knew well my sister and her husband; our way of life was not one cut out for them. They would never understand our dreams, and their concern was sincere.

While in Lima, we were treated in grandeur; nothing was too much for Raul and Vicky who made our stay enjoyable. Sergio and John Paul, not quite six years old, reconnected and became pals again. The following week, well rested, we said goodbye to everyone. Our words of thanks to my sister, her husband, and their friends surely didn't express the depth of our gratitude. We were truly indebted.

The subsequent part of our journey we hoped and prayed would go smoothly, as it would take us through the high Andes Mountains, a treacherous road, before reaching Bolivia.

For the first nine hundred kilometers, we enjoyed the incredible spectacle offered by the Pan-American Highway bordering the Pacific Ocean. Ragged cliffs like concrete walls served as natural retaining walls for the road, while high waves soaring and breaking against it gave us an unparalleled experience of sight and sound, intimidating at times.

Farther south, we found deserted beaches on one side of the road and massive sand dunes on the other. In this arid and deserted region, the motor in the six-ton truck overheated and stopped five hundred kilometers or so before reaching Arequipa, the last place before we went across the mountains, and the city where we planned to replenish groceries, water and gasoline.

It was a used truck to start and it got pushed too hard on the first part of our journey. So here we were, forced to stay put in this forsaken place, only a small village called Chala at a short distance away. John and Walter dismounted the motor and drove to Arequipa to have it fixed.

The rest of us forcefully had to remain put and wait. By the fourth day we had run out of most of our provisions and the locals from the village had only the bare minimum to get on with their own lives. We had thirteen mouths to feed and unfortunately no *Mana* from Moses' time came down to nourish us. So we resorted to the ocean, which had always been a good source; all the males in the group from the youngest to the oldest went fishing and the bounty was good. Not so every day. Those days there was a change in the menu, llama jerky bought from the villagers went into the pot; the salt added to dry the meat camouflaged the wild tang.

The sixth day John and Walter came back with the motor fixed and also brought fresh meat, eggs, milk, and bread; we had a feast! The motor actually had to be rebuilt, the reason for the long wait. Once the motor was back in its niche, the march continued and as planned we stopped in Arequipa to replenish the pantry, and sent a telegraph to my father notifying him that our expected arrival in Cochabamba should take place in close to three days.

On route, John drove the big truck, John Paul and I sat next to him; we had learned our lesson in Mexico. As our convoy started to ascend, the overcast sky brought heavy rain which soon turned to snow causing perilous mudslides along the way. As a precaution, before the real ascent through the Andean mountains began, we decided to have one more overnight stop; it was not safe to travel at night, even more not knowing the treacherousness that lay ahead. Road conditions were not the best, yet because we traveled during the summer season, we felt fairly safe and never expected the horrific experience that followed.

The next morning it was still snowing and as the elevation increased the snow came down more heavily, to the point that when we reached the summit we could not see more than a meter ahead. The altimeter read seventeen thousand feet, which converted into meters, gave the approximate figure of 5.200mts. The caravan moved at a snail's pace and our breathing became laborious; no one had thought to bring any oxygen. Our heads ached as if compacting hammers banged inside our craniums, the children began to vomit and heaved; we all had the runs and bloated abdomens.

In the midst of this nightmare, when we thought it could not get worse, it did. The big truck had a flat tire and the simple routine to change it, became a Herculean effort. In slow motion the frozen bolts were removed, but one broke. The welding equipment had to be brought out; an iron rod was welded transversally and hammered on until the broken bolt was removed; John and Walter took turns, the altitude, the snow and the freezing wind made their endeavors extremely trying, both were physically exhausted.

Prayers kept us collected, although at one point thought we were not going to make it. But I suppose the Lord won't hand you over more than what you can handle, and He must have heard us, because the task was completed and the descent then began. Relief replaced the stress we had lived through the hours before.

Soon Lake Titicaca, the highest one in the world, was in our view together with a bright and warm sun; another day and we would be in Cochabamba. In the next hour we crossed the border town of Puno on the Peruvian side and the *Desaguadero* onto Bolivian soil. As Bolivian officers checked our documents, the nightmare of the last two days was behind us. We felt the same as the Spanish *conquistadores* must have felt hundreds of years ago as they discovered and conquered the land: victorious!

I then saw father approaching. "He is not supposed to be here," I thought and my heart shrank as he came closer. Dad looked bushed, sunken eyes and unshaved, unlike him who always was made up impeccably. He seemed to have aged; the two thought lines between his eyes were deeper. I had not seen my Dad for over four years, true, but his present appearance was more from a person who had not slept in days and had a big worry on his shoulders. Something had to be terribly wrong!

My joy and my present concern, brought tears to my eyes as I embraced my Dad. John shook hands with him and introduced him to our friends. Father after clearing crackling noises from his throat, a symptom that he was very distraught, explained the reason for meeting us at the border. "Two weeks ago the Minister of Agriculture demanded my presence in La Paz. Immediately I flew to meet with him, only to learn that the land granted to your enterprise had been declared a Fiscal Reserve."

I attentively listened to my father's words, not understanding yet the gravity of the situation. Even so, I translated the statement to the rest of the group, including John. The quizzical look on everyone's faces gave Dad the hint we needed a more ample explanation. So he continued, "Fiscal Reserve means that no private enterprise or private persons will own land in that particular area; nor would anyone be allowed to work it. I received the news while you were en route; it was impossible to notify you of this sudden governmental change in time to stop you."

Father was right, how could he have notified us? He didn't know where we might be; neither cell phones, nor e-mails were yet a dream in someone's imagination. The fastest mail was through a regular post; the snail mail way and except for the town of Toluca, in Mexico, we had not made any other arrangements.

The news was devastating! It was not three months ago that the same ministerial office had told my father, "Everything is ready; All we need now is for the group to arrive and sign the final document to finalize the agreement." We left California under that understanding.

Walter and Jean, who had just as much at stake as we did, could not comprehend the absurdity. No one would anyway. In any civilized country something like this would never happen, but then again, in my nation all things were possible. This time it was us who happened to be the sacrificial goats; our beautiful dreams were shattered by the stroke of a Ministerial signature!

Father, our partners and us went back and forth to La Paz, fruit-lessly trying to see the President who had promised to oversee our project, hoping he would personally intervene. However the President was never available. Our struggles continued for the next three months; all fifteen of us were lodged at my parents' house. But the Ministerial change was set and established, no one could intervene now, not even the President.

It was overwhelming and extremely embarrassing for John, my father, and I; we could not just say to our friends, "Sorry guys, these things often happen in Bolivia, but don't take it personally." What a joke. It was very difficult to swallow, even a harder lesson to learn. Our dream ended in a total fiasco.

The business accord with our friends was dissolved and our investment distributed accordingly. Since the core of the money was invested in machinery, equipment, tools and vehicles, all needed to be sold first, which ended at a loss for everyone. A few months later, the other members of our group went back to the States. Not us. John's dream was in Bolivia; he wasn't moving anywhere!

September, 1985

"*Bone Voyage*," I said to Judith, smiling, but after she departed I felt as if I was sitting on pins and needles. I knew her itinerary by heart. In my mind's eye, I envisioned all the check-points she needed to transverse before she was safe at home; I kept my fingers crossed. We had agreed she would call me the moment she arrived, so around that time I didn't allow anyone near the phone while I was expecting her call.

It finally came. Though exhausted, at the same time I was ecstatic; everything had gone as predicted. No one had searched her luggage. All my worries were over for now. Judith promised to call again the moment the deal was completed and had the cash in her hands.

A week went by, then another and another, without a word from her. I could not understand the silence, or the reason for the extended hold up. It was she herself who had distinctly said, "My friend has everything ready." Judith knew I had borrowed the money for the transaction. She was also aware I could have pursued my goal through another contact, so I was disconcerted with her silence.

My patience was at an end. The stress of not knowing what was taking place in France kept me awake at night. I had no doubt in my mind that John Paul's condition was being jeopardized with the delay. Survival rate for AIDS-infected persons had not improved; we were running out of time, even if my son still seemed well.

So I tried to contact her. Several calls later, I talked to her but only to learn that her friend needed more time. I believe fumes came out from my ears when I told Judith to threaten her friend by saying, "You'd better hurry up or Myriam will sell the stuff to someone else!" I thought a bit of pressure would speed up the process.

Judith promised to relay my message, but more time went by and nothing happened. I became ragingly angry as I realized my mistake. I had entrusted Judith and her friend, a couple of amateurs far too much, instead of organizing the deal with Bernard's contact in Spain, and things were piling up on me. Even if my son's condition hadn't deteriorated, he still needed the treatment; plus the money I borrowed from Victor should have been paid back already.

Then an event that should have just brought happiness came, to complicate matters. Sandra, my sister's daughter, was getting married November 10 in Lima. The wedding had been arranged months prior to my crisis and my sister and her husband expected all of us to be there. Vicky had no immediate family in Peru and the ones coming from Bolivia could be counted on the fingers of one hand. What's more, John because of his work would not even be present, neither our younger son Patrick because of his school. Only Mom, John Paul, and I were going.

The delay in France messed everything up. The affair would now have to remain on hold and since I couldn't do anything about it, I made the decision to make the best of the situation and make the trip as part of an enjoyment for John Paul and perhaps even for myself.

My son and his cousin Sergio, brother to the bride, were witnesses at the ceremony. The two were not only cousins they had been pals from the time they were little toddlers. While in Lima,

I was certain Sergio would make sure John Paul had a good time and I appreciated it.

After the ceremony my sister and Raul offered a formal banquet at their home, happy to celebrate this time with their daughter Sandra and her husband, Jaime. The newlyweds left for their honeymoon at midnight, yet most of the guests remained up until dawn. Throughout the wedding and the few days we stayed in Lima, I hid my sorrow to share in my sister's happiness, but my thoughts were in France.

Once back at home, after I checked that John and Patrick were well and had no problems, I called Judith only to learn that my threat to speed up matters had not worked; all I got were more excuses. Nothing made any sense, her explanations were either too far-fetched, or I had become paranoid. I didn't know what to believe anymore; I feared she might have entrusted the cocaine to someone without getting the money in exchange, the reason for her pretext, and didn't even have the courage to tell me the truth.

Harshly I reproached myself, "How could you have been so stupid, to trust them with the sale of the cocaine?" My instinct had failed me; I had approached Judith and accepted the reliability of her friend only because they were part of the social life in Cannes, which I thought gave them the right connections. I now regretted it.

Three and a half months had been wasted. Six, since I first learned of my son's ailment and the bits and pieces publicized in the mass media about AIDS were more disturbing with every day that went by. Every article I read speculated, "Anyone infected, within a year or two at the most, died!"

The political and economic situation in my country was in shambles. I still worked, but I lost interest in the factory since my heart was somewhere else. Internally I agonized and figured the longer the wait the less chance my son had. My hope lay entirely on the findings in France and my anxiety pinnacled because of the failure in closing the French deal.

Insanely, I saw only one way out. If I wanted to complete my objective I had to take other steps, so immediately I sought out Bernard. Leaving all pretenses aside I called him and asked, "Bernard, are you still in touch with your friend in Spain. I need to do business with him." Not waiting for an answer, rudely I kept on with my rhetoric. "How soon can you establish a contact for me, with approximately seven hundred grams?" Cutting in, he replied, "Yes, I'm still in contact with him, Myriam. I can call him right away and I'll let you know his response as soon as possible."

The next day Bernard called me back and I had the answer to my queries, "My friend's name is Mario. He is interested and can be ready to take care of your business right after Christmas, actually December 30th if that date suits you." From the tone of his voice, I detected a smile. "Yes, it certainly does. I'll give you the money in the next day or two. Thanks."

From day one, all I got from Jim and Bernard was help and I appreciated it. I knew I could count on them. I was back in business; at last in a few more weeks I would have the money for my son's treatment. Yet in spite of the good news, I felt frustrated and angry at the failure of my first intent. If Bernard had not lent me a hand again, I would not have been able to do anything to help John Paul.

Obsessed that his life depended on me, I was indifferent to anything else. I didn't even flinch at the thought that I was not only going deeper into debt but also further in the illegal trade; I just closed my eyes and went to see the loan shark again.

The last time I visited him, Victor had left the door open when he said, "If you need more cash, I'll just extend the existing loan, but you will need to keep it in good standing: interests paid, etc." I had indeed kept that part of the deal. So I marched off to see him again, sure he would lend me the extra money. His business was to make a profit, no questions asked, and I was right.

The man was ruthless. Victor must have investigated our assets and found we owned several properties, but was not aware that the house under construction was the only one solely owned by John and I; the rest were joint assets with our business partners Mauricio and his wife. Even so Victor demanded, "I need a mortgage on one of your properties as collateral," he said, smiling while he licked his lips. Supported by what seemed positive presages, I agreed.

Number one, John because of his constant trips had entrusted me with a Power of Attorney to sign business transactions in his absence. Now in total misuse of that trust, without hesitation I put my signature on the contract.

Secondly my in-laws in Canada, who wanted to see their son over Christmas but knew that a trip of this nature presently was out of our reach, decided to pay for John's tickets themselves. Their largesse was superb. He certainly needed a break, besides that there invite fitted very well with my own plans. John's time away from home would give me the freedom I needed and no call for explanations!

In a flash something else came to my mind and told my husband, "Honey, why don't you ask your parents to include Patrick in their plans? He missed the trips J. P. and I took because of his schooling. If Patrick goes with you, he will have the opportunity to strengthen the relationship with his Canadian grandparents and at the same time have some fun too. I'm sure they won't mind paying for his tickets as well. Nana will love to see him again. What do you think?" My husband was all for it and his parents graciously accepted his request.

If that was not enough, a third mind-boggling incident happened. Our partner Mauricio, who never before had taken time off from the factory, chose this particular time to spend the holiday season with his family in the United States. His oldest daughter and son attended a university in Baltimore. Mauricio's decision could not have come at a better moment; no explanations needed for him either.

Three great phenomena were in motion, and none were set up by me; all too encouraging since the part played by Judith was on the rocks. It proved to me that the way was opened again for my mission to succeed.

John and Patrick left for Canada December 22; their intention was to stay for a month, more than enough time for me to complete my own journey. John Paul had no idea of any of my brewing or for that matter of any of my misgivings. I knew he had just conformed to his destiny. Not I!

For his benefit I elaborated a pretty credible tale. "Judith has obtained a large contract for Bolivian artisan's goods, in llama and alpaca. In order to sign the deal, I'll need to go for a short while to France with samples and catalogues.

Suddenly another idea came to my mind that immediately I voiced to J. P. in a question form, smiling, "Would you like to come along John Paul? Once I conclude the business, we'll go together to Paris. I believe Judith has already some advance money," I lied.

My smile was a fake, my excitement too; nonetheless I had to perform the best act of my life to make him believe me. With more legroom to operate now, the impulse to take him along with me had just popped up at the last minute; therefore my story had to be flawless.

It was important that John Paul would not put any resistance to my invitation. I figured that once I got the money in Spain, it was best my son was with me, so that we could continue together to Paris and get on with the treatment. To give my fib a genuine appearance, I even bought an assortment of alpaca samples and some catalogues

My son, who still had the taste from the trip before said, "Oh, Mom that would be awesome. Are you serious?" he asked me is disbelief. "Sure I am serious.

BOLIVIA, 1967

IT TOOK A WHILE BEFORE JOHN FOUND A JOB, BUT HIS ENGINEERING background opened doors. Contracted as a Consultant Engineer in a variety of projects, my husband was soon a well recognized professional, and Bolivia became our permanent home, which made me incredibly happy. I was near to all that was dear to me: my parents, my friends, plus the Bolivian lifestyle with my country's specialties cuisine. I felt like a fish in water and so did John.

John Paul at first missed the Martin clan, but he soon leaped into the new plan. The relationship he had earlier on with his grandfather, as a toddler was now more profound; our son looked to his grandpa as another mentor. Enrolled in first grade at the *Colegio Loyola,* an excellent Catholic elementary school for boys and girls, John Paul soon had many friends.

Everything fell into place like pieces of a beautiful puzzle and in no time John and I had a group of compatible friends: couples with children who the same as us enjoyed the outdoor life. My cousin Raul and his wife Lila were among them. They had come back to Bolivia a couple of years earlier and now had seven children. Ramiro, a civil engineer and his wife Isabella, had six. Mauricio and Betty had five. These three couples were our most assiduous friends and John Paul, who was still our only child, could not get enough of their children when we all got together; yet he could also be just as contented playing on his own.

I had known Mauricio all my life. Striving and ambitious, he now owned a small marble and tile manufacturing plant. John and Mauricio got along well. Having great aspirations, he let my husband know, "My goal is to expand the plant; but I haven't yet the credit rapport with banking entities to ask for a loan for my project.

"There is an open market for all the products we manufacture and the services we provide; I'm sure the demand will increase. I expect a growth of at least 200 % per year, but I need capital to put my plan into practice. Would you be interested in investing with me, John?"

My husband saw the potential in Mauricio's initiative and also eager to spread out his wings asked his new friend, "How much would you need Mauricio?" He apparently had summarized his needs ahead of time, and quickly responded. "Not much, ten thousand dollars will do and you'll have fifty percent in the partnership."

The venture was still in development and had all the struggles any new industry brought along, but John after a short exchange of opinions with me, accepted. We had just finished liquidating the rest of the equipment left from our previous venture and he invested the proceeds with my old friend.

From the start my husband never questioned or intervened in any of the factory decisions; he totally trusted his comrade's vision. Mauricio alone oversaw every aspect of the company. He imported, at a high cost, marble slabs from Argentina and had six or eight workers who assembled the pieces and polished the mosaics. John's investment went to purchase specific machinery to cut into slabs the Bolivian marble brought in by blocks.

Early on *campesinos* from different regions brought a variety of samples, of onyx, travertine, black and dark green marbles, rudimentarily extracted, damaged by the dynamite used in the exploitation. John took interest and taught the same peasants better methods of extraction and in no time they brought marble blocks in excellent condition.

The factory no longer needed to import marble, thus prices of the products dropped and clients began to abound. I had been assisting Mauricio on a part-time basis until then, but as it expanded I went into full-time. The partnership's ultimate goal was the success of the enterprise, so any profit made was re-invested back into the factory.

About our love life, everything was hanky dory, as John would say. Yet we still had only one offspring. We had been back in my city for the past two years and married for eight. It just didn't happen. When still in foreign lands, often my husband would bring up the subject and I teasingly used to respond, "Honey if we stay away from my country, one child is more than I can handle. Looking after you, John Paul, the house, the cooking, and my work; I don't think I can handle anything more. "

John would frown thinking I was serious, when in reality I was only joking. The disconcerted look on his face was pitiful, so I playfully added. "Don't worry sweetheart; the problem can be easily solved; if you want we could have a dozen but only if you take me back to Bolivia." He then burst out laughing at my perspective.

But there was no sign of at least one more child out of the dozen I had promised we would have. Worried, I'd visited a specialist who placed me under a fertility program which did not appear to be working.

February 24th 1969, I had my bi-weekly visit with the gynecologist. The same day my Dad's physician had asked me to stop by his office too. For some unknown reason he wanted to see me alone, without my father.

The request was unusual and I was a bit nervous. My nervousness turned into disbelief as I listened to the doctor's words, "I'm sorry to have to tell you Myriam, but I must. Your father has cancer of the lymph nodes. The prognosis is not good because of the nature of the cancer; it has spread. He might have only six more months to live."

"No, I don't believe you. My father is fine, he hasn't been ill; how can you entertain even the possibility that he has cancer?" Angered and tearful I refuted the doctor's diagnosis. "Sorry Myriam but your father does have cancer. I wanted to be totally certain before I broke the news to you, the reason why I re-tested him several times. It has now been confirmed."

Numbed by the blow I was unable to think straight. My father had been my rock and my hero in my growing up years, as a matter of fact all through my life. I could not lose him. I knew father had not felt that well, but I thought it was nothing serious. I never expected to hear otherwise. I agreed with the doctor it was best to momentarily keep the news from my father and mother; it could only accelerate his collapse.

Brokenhearted I went to see my own doctor, who for the past year had been checking me for results on my treatment. Not mentally there, I heard the OB/GYN say, "Myriam you are pregnant!" His words didn't sink in yet, but when they did I asked, "What? It can't be. Last time I was here you forewarned me that the treatment was not working. I'm really pregnant? Are you serious?" It had to be a miracle! Early on, because of the problems I was having, the gynecologist had advised me to have a hysterectomy. Only thanks to my stubbornness that had not happened.

Our second son was born on October 16, 1969, christened a week later as Patrick Ivan: handsome and powerful names. Monsignor Walter Rosales, a dear friend of the family celebrated the ceremony and my father and John Paul were Patrick's godparents. It was J. P. who requested to share this responsibility with his grandfather; he was always surprising us with his maturity and assuming responsibilities beyond his years. Our first son was nine years old and the dream of his short little life had always been to have a sibling. He never wanted to be the only child and finally his wish had come true.

Patrick's first three years however were a pure struggle for survival. His health was so fragile that he was constantly under the care of specialized pediatricians. We had two terrifying experiences when we almost lost him. Later he outgrew all of his health problems and though still a slim child, he was otherwise strong and healthy.

January 11, 1973, we suffered the loss of my father. He died at home. My mother, my husband and I were by his bedside; Vicky, who a month earlier had come from Lima was by his side as well. The funeral was magnificent. He was given full military honors. This was a great source of pride for us, but it didn't alleviate the irreparable sense of loss we felt. For John Paul who was only twelve years old, the loss of his grandfather was hard to bear; he had been very close to him. Patrick was still too young to feel the grief.

As for myself, after his passing my heart hardened. I had seen his suffering; a whole three years. I had lived through it. The sorrow of death had not touched me before as my grandparents were gone before I was even born. My father's death became personal. When he died, a part of me died as well and I began to dissociate from God.

Bolivia had gone through a period of political and economic instability up until 1971, when through a *coup d'état* an army General took over the government. A dictatorship was initiated, and good, bad or indifferent, it brought back political tranquility, bolstering the Bolivian economy.

A new era of economic bonanza dawned in the country and in our factory as well. Sales took off. It allowed us to purchase two lots in one of the most fashionable subdivision in town. Three months later, in chain reaction, the construction of our homes began; Mauricio's was completed first months, ours followed shortly after.

The new homes were beautiful, but I found ours a little too elaborate. Mauricio had intervened in the finishing touches. Soon I learned our friend liked to do things his way, or no way! My husband, easy going as usual, didn't care. He generally didn't take part in any of the business decisions. Often away from home, on field trips, he completely trusted my judgment as well as Mauricio's and left everything in our hands.

The architectural design of our house was superb; it was the interior detail which bothered me. A bit too much marble, not enough hardwood, I suppose I could have lived with it, but the wallpaper was too bright and colorful; the thought I would have to reside there was driving me insane. Why didn't I just say to Mauricio, "I don't like it." I suppose because neither John nor I wanted to openly complain.

Feelings get too easily hurt and Mauricio in that sense was very touchy. It was best not to bring the subject up, but in a round about way I approached our partner with another technique, "Mauricio a while back we talked about one day building custom homes, remember?" I let him nibble on that thought with a big smile before continuing, "We even discussed how great it would be to break into this field when we had the money, do you follow me?"

"So, what about it?" Mauricio responded flatly. Encouragingly I smiled again and said, "Well don't you think right now could be the right time?" I wasn't about to give up. My plan had to work. "So, do we rob a bank for the money?" His response didn't open any doors. He certainly was not cooperating in this conversation.

"No, we don't need to clobber a banker to get the money; how about if we sell my house, it's already built. It will give us the start up capital. John, the kids, and I, we can still stay at my mother's house for a while. I'm sure she won't mind." I was not too sure about the quizzical look Mauricio gave me, while he processed everything.

At last he said, "Okay, okay, you are right. It's a good time to put my idea into practice." He had come to terms. The initiative was his now and very thoughtfully he asked me, "Are you sure? Do you really want to give up your house Myriam?" I didn't say it out loud; I just nodded, while inside I shouted, *yes of course!*

By now I knew Mauricio's ways fairly well. I learned that if I wanted to put something of my own in practice, I had to do it indirectly. Our partner did wonders if the idea was his. So for the sake of peacekeeping, I developed this tactic to the point it was an art, otherwise our partnership would have been a battlefield.

Our house sold a month later at an excellent price. Tickled with excitement, I told John and Mauricio, "Lets have a party; we need to celebrate this occasion." I didn't see the response I expected, so to steer them to my level, I added, "Can you image the promotion it will give to our new construction business, and even more for our marble products?"

That did it. Actually John was all for it from the moment I opened my mouth. He always backed me up in whatever plans I had; he was convinced I had a good business mind. My aim was to interest Mauricio, so we could all work together towards the success of both ventures, the factory, and of our new construction company: my baby. Mauricio liked the idea and accepted it. After all, the place was a good showcase.

The list of guests was long; my dowry to my marriage and to the partnership was an unlimited amount of friends in places of high power, political as well as other ranks. The new owners of the house were invited, as well as the Mayor of our city, the Minister of Finance, who was in town from La Paz, bank managers, and certainly our regular friends, all with their female counterparts, of course.

Mario and his wife Lucia were first n our list. He was a party person himself and a good dancer and just because he presently was my husband's boss in a huge hydroelectric project was not enough reason to leave him out.

Once I got the okay, we all went overboard to make the party a success. Solely for the occasion we had the house professionally decorated and furnished; again friends gave us a hand. The beautiful bouquets of flowers sent by our guests, placed in different areas of the house gave an even greater grandeur to the full décor.

Mauricio's wife prepared an exquisite buffet supper; Betty always excelled in the culinary art.

John's domain was the bar; he had a complete assortment of cocktails and drinks ready for the night. Some of our loyal factory workers, who also wanted to participate in the celebration, came dressed in blue pants, white shirts and bow ties to help us; they became professional waiters and bartenders for the night and did an outstanding job.

Incidentally, it was my birthday as well. Rose, the company's bookkeeper, on her own accord brought a group of Mariachis dressed in their typical Mexican costumes to be part of the bash. They provided much of the entertainment as they marched in singing the Happy Birthday; from that point on, the party really got started.

Everyone danced, dined, and drank to their hearts content until dawn. The party turned into a great success; it was talked about for a long time afterwards, unquestionably the beginning of my stardom.

Mauricio always prided himself saying, "The only business advertisement our company needs is the beautiful end results we create with the marble." Nothing was more true. Yet John and I added our two cents too. Entertaining clients as well as bank officials, was another key ingredient for our success. We did a lot of that.

Soon the factory's new structure was completed and the manufacturing plant relocated. It allowed us to undertake greater and more profitable contracts. The financial institutions, seeing our efforts as a young industry aimed at doing well, opened up loans and new credit lines. The opportunity to diversify into another arena, fell in our lap. We purchased a large parcel of land, to later develop as an exclusive subdivision.

We also bought a lot, half a block away from Mauricio's place, where our new home would be built; all happening within a year after the sale of our house! John Paul, fourteen now, was delegated by John and I to sketch the initial drawings. He already had proven his exceptional artistic abilities. We all participated, even Patrick; we brought ideas to the table and J.P. the interpreter drew it, and *voilà*, we had the outline of an incredible split level rancher of about four thousand square feet. At the back of the house, the maid's quarters, the laundry room, the garden shed and space for a possible swimming pool.

In business matters everything went through Mauricio before it proceeded to the next step; understandable, after all, as he was the initiator of the venture and the general manager. So now without a second thought our house's sketch followed the same course; our partner made a few corrections and being that Mauricio also had a formidable architectural vision, he penciled in the roof.

The final drawings were signed off by an architect then went to the Municipality for the building permit. Under Mauricio's supervision our beautiful home began to take shape.

December, 1985

Gustavo, the owner of the travel agency knew us well. He had no problem to issue the two round trip tickets to France. At my request he agreed to bill us the three thousand dollars owing at the end of the month. After all we were good clients.

My existing debt pile grew, but I didn't flinch. To get my son to Paris quickly was all that mattered. I had it well figured out; even that once I concluded my business in Spain, I would open an account in US currency in Paris for John Paul to have access to the money and I could just slip back to Cochabamba.

My short absence would not be noticed by anyone. My mother satisfied with my tale that I was going to Brazil to purchase a car, didn't bother to ask any other questions. Rose again was the sole person who knew the true nature of my trip and she agreed to cover for me at the factory.

A few days before our departure, I had a phone call from George, who ask me, "If you still have in mind to send John Paul to France, I have some information that might help in the search. He then recalled my attention to a childhood friend whom currently resided in Spain. "Remember Luis José Boero? He is a renowned doctor in Barcelona. He likely has connections with colleagues in the medical profession in France. I have his phone number, would you like to have it?" "Of course George," I replied.. "I remember

Luis José very well. It's wonderful he has attained recognition in Spain. It couldn't be otherwise; he was so smart. I'll call him right away. Thank you for the information."

The moment Luis José heard my distress, told me, "Myriam I'll be happy to help you. I'll have a letter ready for a friend of mine. He is a specialist in blood disorders in Paris. If he can't help your son himself, I'm sure he will refer him to some one else who will. Call me the minute you are in Barcelona. I'll guide you then in how to get to my place."

"That is awesome Luis José. I'll do just that; see you soon and thanks." To learn about him and that he practiced and resided in Barcelona came as another unexpected boost; except for Judith's malfunctioning deal, all the other good stuff proved more than ever that I was doing only what was right!

On Christmas day I called John to wish him and Patrick, as well as his parents, a Merry Christmas. While I was on the phone the faint voice of my conscience gave me a piece of advice, "You can't just go to France, leaving your husband and Patrick in complete ignorance as to your whereabouts?" So producing the same lie I fabricated for J.P., I told him, "Judith has an important purchase order for our export-import business in France. I have to go there to sign the contract."

It was all very plausible, but I added something just as reasonable for John Paul's trip and for the time he might need to remain in France for the treatment, "John Paul is coming with me; he has the opportunity to work again with Judith as a tourist guide" John accepted my explanations without question. He was actually excited with the news and happy with our good fortune.

With everything pretty much in place, the day before our flight I called Judith to let her know I was on my way to France. I had given up hope about her; my call was only to ask her if she could lodge us for a day or two. While making my point, she surprised me; "My friend has the contact ready. She will close the deal any time now." It was a relief to learn my worries had been unfounded; she had not lost the drug, but it was too late to change my plans.

Impossible to retrace my steps, I could not give back the recently purchased cocaine, nor tell my husband and John Paul that our trip to France was canceled; all my lies would be out in the open! My only option was to continue with my most recent plan. Once in France, I would sell the fourteen hundred grams of cocaine and be done with it.

Unable to contain my annoyance, I told her, "You have no idea the stress your friend's excuses and later your lengthy silence caused me. I thought something had gone wrong with the deal. I've actually purchased more of the stuff. You knew I needed the money right now, not in a hundred years. I don't understand the delay or your silence?"

She tried to interrupt, but I continued, "I have someone reliable now. Someone I know well," I lied to make my next sentence sound stronger. "I'll be in France December 27th around nine in the morning; all I need from you now is a place to stay. I'll pick up the stuff I entrusted to you and the problem will no longer be yours."

Judith, not happy with my decision, argued, "You're being unfair. I believe we deserve another chance. Particularly since my friend has tried so hard to find a contact." The moment she said those words, I cut her short, "For starters, your friend told you, 'I'll have everything set and ready for your arrival.' Was she not telling the truth then? It's beside the point now anyway. I will give you the chance you want if you think she will close the deal with no more delays. You can go ahead. You have my blessing."

Judith immediately said, "She will, don't worry." Changing the subject I added, "By the way, I need you to back me up in something; John Paul is coming with me. I don't want you to mention anything in front of him; if you have to say something just say, 'The Alpaca business is going great,' and agree with me to whatever else I talk about, okay? I'll explain everything later."

December 27th 1985 John Paul and I boarded a plane for France, via Miami, New York, a short touch down in Paris. and our trip ending in Nice. The 700grms of cocaine in my suitcase.

Even though broken inside, an outward look was vital for me, no matter the circumstances. So I wore my best mid-season outfit: charcoal trousers and jacket, a red blouse, completed with a well-tailored coat, black leather boots, purse and gloves. John Paul dressed in a pair of tan pants, the same color turtle neck jersey, a dark brown sport leather jacket that matched the color of his shoes, both looking as if we just had stepped out from a magazine. After all we were heading for Europe.

Once aboard the plane, John Paul strangely intuitive asked, "Mom is everything okay? You seem a bit odd." Smiling I shook my head and said, "I'm fine." J.P unsatisfied with my brief answer, asked again, "I still think there is something strange about this trip; I know you are determined I seek the help from doctors in France, but are you sure there is nothing conflictive in this whole thing?"

My abrupt decision to bring J.P. along on the trip was a good enough reason to give some concern to my son, even more if he had detected my tension. I have to control my nerves better, I thought, while I also saw necessary to be more explicit with my answers. J.P. didn't need to worry.

"No John Paul, everything is okay. I've already explained to you. First I've business to attend to in Nice. After, I intend to go to Barcelona to meet with my friend, Luis José, the doctor...remember I told you about him? He has promised to help us. He'll give us a referral letter for an excellent colleague in Paris. His reference will open some doors and make matters easier in our search.

"If I'm nervous it is because I wish we were already there! And no, I'm not doing anything wrong. Why would you ask me such a thing, anyway?" As if nothing troubled me I responded with an innocent look on my face and continued talking about other topics. My son seemed at ease now, anticipation coming all through his pores and why not? We were en route to France to find the cure for his illness.

Miami was our first stop; we knew this airport very well as South American travelers with connecting flights to other cities or countries, inevitably had to go through Miami, where a systematic luggage inspection was in place. I didn't expect it to be any different this time.

While I marched with John Paul to retrieve our suitcases I looked unshaken externally, but internally my heart was ready to explode. I prayed no one would notice that as we continued forward to the custom checkout counters, to the one designated to us according to an assigned color. Red meant complete inspection of the suitcases, yellow not as a thorough scrutiny, but just the same the luggage had to be opened; luck was on my side as a green light blinked and John Paul and I went by Customs with our suitcases untouched.

The next stop in our itinerary came next, New York. Once up in the air, John Paul who liked to watch movies asked me if I wanted to see one, but too worn out from all the hustle, I declined.

The wine I had with supper had sent me in to a nostalgic mood, so closing my eyes I wandered off to a different time zone, a happy one in another era. I evoked our trips to the *Chapare;* a tropical region only two and half-hours drive from Cochabamba, where John, our two sons and I often went. Just for the day sometimes, others in camping trips with a group of friends we used to hang around for entire weekends

The rivers had crystalline waters, with swift currents and spectacular swimming holes. Everyone from age one to sixty enjoyed the recreation this paradise provided. Villa Tunari the province's city and capital, offered other treats too. It came in a culinary form; all we could eat of the most delicious fish called *surubi*, with crispy fried yucca, or in a delicious soup, served under palm huts or banana trees.

A trip to Villa Tunary necessarily involved passing through Shinahota, a town a few kilometers before; well known for the quantity of coca growers; the process of preparing a cocaine base came later and involved *campesinos*. I suppose for them it was just a way of making a living. At the time it was still a friendly place, but not too reputable.

Villa Tunary was a tropical paradise, and what ever was going on in Shinahota, didn't stop the flow of people, nor us. We just avoided the area and zoomed by passing the town to whichever swimming hole we chose for the occasion.

What a paradox it was that I now carried in my suitcase that stuff made by those *campesinos*, but refined by my new friend José, the chemist! Returning into the past had helped me relax, but also made me wonder about the incredible loops life plays in our lives.

July, 1976

"Honey, ten years have gone by since the day we first set foot on Bolivian soil as courageous *Conquistadors*, it is now time to take a break and visit my parents," John said and waited a moment to see my reaction. Surprised, I didn't say anything yet.

We all certainly needed a vacation; he was right and to go to Canada right again. John Paul was only five when he last saw his grandparents and Patrick had not even met them. Our sons were fifteen and six now, an excellent time to reconnect with the other part of their heritage and start a relationship with their Canadian grandparents.

While building our future, we just could not handle the expenses, but now we could easily afford the cost of a trip to Canada; in the past ten years we'd prospered!

As if reading my thoughts John happily continued, "I'm sure Mauricio can manage without you for a while. John Paul's term year ends in a couple of weeks, Patrick is off from school for his winter break; we can even take your mother with us."

His grin grew sure that all he said was setting very well with me and added something else yet more interesting, "Miami is a necessary stop on our way to Canada and you mentioned we still need some things, such as appliances and other décor for our new home. We can purchase those items at wholesale outlets in Miami and no sales tax would be added to our bill; it will represent great saving for us, dear." That did it; we were going shopping!

John told Mauricio our plans. He was happy for us, but perhaps a little disappointed that he was not able do something similar with his family.

My mother, invited by John agreed to join us under one condition, "I'll love to come, but only if you let me pay the plane tickets to Miami and back." Her generous bargain of course was accepted, which now initiated another idea. "We could buy a vehicle in Miami and continue the trip to Calgary by car." John said, happy with this new option. "It will give our sons new experiences; a tiny taste of the life we had before we came back to Bolivia; the travels, the explorations, and the fun."

My husband brought that adventurous look into his face, which was all too familiar to me as he continued putting his ideas in front of a very attentive audience: John Paul and Patrick. The boys listened and didn't let their father say another word, in unison shouting, "Let's do it, let's go for it, Dad!" And off we went

Once in Miami, we found a conveniently located motel, pool included, then unloaded our luggage and went shopping. SUVs were not around yet, but the fairly new but used Pontiac Mark III we purchased matched the present utility models.. Six people could comfortably seat in it, and we were only five. The large trunk held our suitcases, a tent, sleeping bags and the rest of the paraphernalia acquired for the planned expedition.

The serious shopping came next: appliances, wall-to-wall carpets, wallpaper, curtains, lamps, linens, etc., and all the stuff we needed for our new home, bought from wholesale outlets at half of what it would have cost us back home. We left the handling and shipping to a broker and light weighted we continued our trip as tourists. First stop: Disney World.

For the next three days we set up camp in a nearby campsite and as soon as the park doors opened until they closed, roller-coasters, submarines and flying saucers rides were the menu of the day, and in between that, variety shows. Mom and I didn't jump aboard on all the rides; some were too extreme. We chose instead to stay put seated under the shade of a tree and found other just as amusing entertainment; we watched the multitude of people walking by us, some who apparently had not restrained themselves in their eating habits.

We had a wonderful taste of this fantasyland, but the main objective of our travel was to get to Canada as fast as we could. Consequently, even though we took the scenic route bordering the Atlantic Ocean, or close to it, we left behind numerous states unexplored. Motels were a welcome accommodation if a well-rested night was needed for the next day's travel. If on the contrary we fancied a site and wanted to enjoy the fun it provided, our tent was set up for a day or two.

Washington, DC had many points of significance to offer, so that is exactly what we did, though certainly not on the foot steps of the White house. No, we found the right campsite close enough and like busy bees we zoomed through all the areas of interest: Capitol Hill, The Smithsonian National museum, Jefferson's and Lincoln's Memorials, the Arlington National Cemetery. Summer was in place and with the weather in our side, every place we stopped filled all our expectations and beyond, but a race against time pushed us to move on.

We whizzed through more eastern states heading north; the Pontiac seemed to have turned into a flying saucer, and an invisible one at that because no police cruiser caught up with us. Soon United States of America was left behind and we were in Ottawa, the starting point of instruction on the other half of our son's heritage; both boys had dual citizenships and it was important to broaden their knowledge about their Dad's origin.

The plan was to visit Parliament Hill, the House of Commons, and of course Canadian museums, but as we arrived we found the city fully dressed; Canadian flags were everywhere and a solemn parade in progress. It happened to be the 1st of July, Canada Day; we had lost track of time along the way. We quickly made a change of plans and sat to watch the parade. We later took a ride around the historical monuments.

Then came the famous Metro Toronto Zoo in Toronto where we spent a few hours; well worth it, the same as Niagara Falls. The falls on the Canadian side were breath taking, however we needed to continue forward.

As we drove through the next towns we had another type of excitement, John's family name, plus first names still used by some family members were inscribed in places of recognition. My husband was aware of the existence of this region, but had never visited it himself. John's ancestors from his father's side had come from Scotland and England as settlers and had made history in their path. Some parks as well as streets were named after them, a cause of great pride for our sons and us.

The Great Lakes in Ontario went by. Magnificent, blue waters on one side and on the other verdant woodland, but soon this beautiful forest became endlessly tedious. The never-ending mass of pine trees mixed with maples, oaks and elms continued through Manitoba. Gradually it changed; not dramatically, just with shorter pine trees mixed with poplars and willows now. Amazingly John Paul and Patrick, always eager to see and learn more were the best of travelers. We never heard a word of complaint during this extremely long journey, or used the commonly question asked by children these days, "Are we there yet?"

Other than that by now we had all begun to feel the strain of being cooped up inside the car, no matter how big or comfortable it was. We all wanted to get there, and fast. After hours of seeing the same type of landscape, an adjustment in the scenery was urgent. So very eloquently and almost simultaneously we all said to John, "Isn't this forest ever going to end, it's too boring!"

Before he had chance to respond, it ended as we entered the Saskatchewan prairies. A welcome change until we found ourselves in a never-ending sea of wheat fields on both sides of the road. By now the drag of the long stretches of the Canadian highways had us all thrashed. Canada covered an immense territory!

Supposedly, we were getting closer. At this point, all of us except for John wondered if we really were getting closer to anything? Or if we would be forever wandering in the Canadian territory, like Moses rambled in the desert. It was around this area, we had to check out a very special land mark, Loverna, the town where John spent his early childhood years. It was a place that brought beautiful memories to his heart, where he was born and lived with his mother and brother at his grandparents' house after his father died.

As we headed southwest, supposedly closer to the Alberta border, unexpectedly John detoured from the main road, nothing in sight except more wheat fields. My husband, who after all these many years seemed to know where he was going, veered to the right, a side road, still paved which soon turned into gravel, then continued into a dirt one that suddenly was just a trail. A couple of hundred meters later, the path disappeared altogether and all we had in front of us was a massive field of wheat.

We could not help but started to laugh and crack jokes seeing the spectacle, "We are now totally lost aren't we Dad? Would you like to use my compass?" John Paul spoke offering the instrument to his Dad. I followed suit by saying, "I thought you said you knew where you were going. I don't see your grandparents house. Where is it, dear?"

Even our little Patrick, sweetly placed his opinion, "Dad, don't you think we should turn back. I don't think we'll be able to find your grandparents' place." John just ignored our unsolicited comments. My mother was the only one with enough sense to keep silent. John certainly didn't turn around, or back. He stubbornly continued driving through the wheat field, and what a surprise we all had!

John knew all along where he was going, but Loverna had turned into a ghost town. Only two houses remained standing, one being his grandparents' former home which, supposedly was very spacious, had provided comfort for the entire family. The general store was in a building next door: the only one for miles around. Yet my husband stared at the house in a state of disbelief. We didn't understand why.

Past memories and curiosity gave us the nerve to ask the present owners to allow us to see it at close range. It was well kept, but John's problem was that he couldn't understand what happened to the size...the huge house he remembered from his childhood had shrunk!

Next we stopped at the cemetery, where his Dad and other deceased family members were buried and we were greatly surprised that the place was unbelievably well kept, not a weed in sight.

With this part of the mission accomplished, John turned around and headed for the Rocky Mountains, our stomping grounds a few years back. From Banff we called his parents to assure them we were still on track, only two hours away. The minute we arrived the excitement and the laughter began, everyone talking at the same time, and no one making too much sense. We were just happy to be together again!

John's parents were pleased to meet my mother, but focused their attention on our sons. They had not seen John Paul since he was an infant and Patrick was the grandson they had never met. He was now Nana's boy. The boys were thrilled to have that much attention from their Canadian grandparents was a treat. Immediately they became official interpreters for their two grand-mothers, who without them, didn't understand a word of what the other one said, but kept on talking, getting along splendidly.

Later John's brother Kenneth, his wife Kay, and their family joined us. The moment could not have been any greater. We knew his two oldest ones, Sue and Kenny; they were a bit older than J.P. Yet only now we met the younger ones, Amy and Heather, who were just a little older than Patrick.

It was an awesome family reunion, unfortunately the two weeks planned with them passed by too quickly. Our time had been cut too short; we had only four days to cover thousands of kilometers to return to Miami and catch our plane back to Bolivia.

As we were leaving, John's parents and Kenneth promised, "We'll work on the next visit, but it will be by plane not by land," they clarified laughing.

We were more pressed for time than ever, yet as we drove through Yellowstone National Park it was impossible to ignore the temptation; we had to see the geysers blast in the air, especially Old Faithful. We understood she was always on time, yet because we got there late for her hourly presentation, we had to wait one more hour before she made her next great appearance. Satisfied with the scene, we drew a diagonal line towards Florida with no more stops, except for fuel and tummy refills as well as some potty breaks.

We made it back in time and arranged the quick sale of our car. We got the same price we paid, and boarded the plane back to Bolivia. At the airport, Mauricio waited for us; had a big smile on his face while he greeted us, which faded away the minute I jokingly said, "Dear Mauricio, I'm exhausted. I need another vacation to recuperate from this one." He laughed a little, but I don't think he appreciated my joke!

It was good to resume our daily routine; better yet to see that our house was completed. It only needed the finishing touches, the ones soon to arrive from Miami. This time our home turned out not only exquisite but also relaxed, exactly the way I wanted.

By the end of September we moved in. Daisy the housekeeper, at my mother's service for some years, came with us. With our businesses on the rise, I was now Mauricio's right arm, and my time was captured by my work. Frequently called to sign contracts or to oversee the work in different cities, I would set off for a day or two. John sometimes was also gone on field trips, and in our absences Daisy's dedication ensured all our son's needs were met.

As a Consulting Engineer for the National Power Company on joint projects with the United Nations, John's time away from home was not as lengthy anymore. Yet he was happy to leave the running of both enterprises entirely in Mauricio's hands and mine. Except for the hospitality side of the deal, in which John was an expert and loved to do together with me.

Our new home was perfect to entertain clients as well as friends, and soon we were engaged in more company parties. Everyone who came to our gatherings enjoyed the soirees, not only because of the good food served but also for the unlimited consumption of alcohol.

Even so, we never failed to provide our sons with our love and attention. Their friends were always welcome at our home, more often than not for overnight visits. Parties organized by J.P.'s class took place at our home, the same as Patrick's Boy Scouts' meetings; it was our preference. John and I were happier having a household full of youngsters than having our sons spend time elsewhere. I took great pride in the relationship we had with our two sons.

However the higher the climb in the business world, the easier it became for me to look the other way to stuff that not to long ago I would have disapproved of, at home and elsewhere. Such as during John Paul's last high school year, I noticed him smoking marijuana. Not openly, nor much, but I didn't confront him; I simply ignored it.

J. P. himself, sure his brother was not around, sheepishly put the question in front of me, "Mom, did you know I smoke marijuana?" "No. Do you?" pretending I didn't know, I responded. "I'll tell you Mom, I prefer to smoke marijuana than the cigarettes you and Dad smoke. Confronted now with the fact, I didn't make any fuss. I appreciated his trust instead. In my view my son had no faults and smoking pot was nothing to worry about it.

What's more I found it foolish to veto it, knowing that it might only make him react negatively. Like some other young people I knew who smoked and drank behind their parents' backs In this aspect, John and I thought alike. We didn't want our sons have the urge to try something, simply because it was forbidden. Instead, sometimes invited by us, J. P. joined us for a drink or two. We didn't see any reason why not; he was about to graduate. Likely all wrong, our life style had so gradually changed that we didn't realize that it was taken us in a down hill road.

Graduation day came, and what a rewarding moment for John and I to see our son receive his diploma. John Paul's interest had always been more in the field of arts, so to end high school with all the curriculum completed was a great accomplishment. We were proud of our son.

In the evening the graduates, with our consent, threw a bash in our home; they danced to the tune of a live band, ate what Daisy and I prepared and drank from the stash that John had in the cooler. Some parents, invited by us, came to celebrate the occasion in grand style as well.

A traditional reward arranged by the school entourage came right after. The alumnae chose a trip to Lima, which entailed going to Machu Picchu as well, the Inca ruins in Cuzco; of course it was all paid for by the parents. After his return, still excited from the expedition, our son mentioned his plans to continue into higher studies. However Bolivian universities were constantly disrupted by political strikes and offered only uncertainties. If teachers were not promoting one, students would decide to have strike on their own; it was very discouraging for young people trying to seek a career.

Realizing the problem will just continue, I discussed a possible solution with my husband, "I don't think John Paul's studies stand a chance here, with all the strikes and subversions happening at the universities. Teachers and students have their own agenda and the problem won't ever be solved. We have to find better options for our son; I believe we should send J.P. to California where he can secure an academic career without the aggravation. What do you think, honey?"

John who had listened quietly considering the pros and cons of my suggestion questioned, "Myriam, can we afford such an outflow? Universities in the States are costly, besides the cost of housing, food, books and the other miscellaneous expenses that John Paul will require?"

My husband normally didn't get involved in the managing aspect of our finances, therefore at this point he didn't know where we stood financially. His earnings, which were excellent, got directly deposited in our joint account, the same happened with the money I withdrew from the factory in salary and dividends; end of the story. Only if John had an investment in mind, like a gold mine, or something else, would he ask me for figures.

The country's economy had continue been on the rise, and both our businesses were running ferociously well. The demand for our products now extended to other cities, the factory contracts had multiplied and the customized homes built by our construction company, sold the minute they were finished. The generated profits were poured back into the two industries, yielding incredibly good returns.

Now our son's future had to be weighed. It had to be thought out together, even if lately John had allowed me take many decisions on my own. "I believe we can manage the expenses, John," I said showing him the numbers. He examined the paper and once he saw the state of our financial affairs was sound, my husband agreed it was a good plan.

This was an incredible act of bravado on my part, not because of the money issue, no. John Paul because of his father's absences had always been my companion from a very young age. As he became older I often consulted family and business matters with him; this time away from us would create a terrible void for me. In spite of this, I saw the significance to provide our son access to a more solid ground for his professional future and John shared in my view.

Once we had all summed up, we made our son aware of the new plan. John Paul, thrilled with the news, could not restrain himself and with teary eyes said, "You are the greatest parents in the world. All along I wanted to study Fine Arts but as you know the Bolivian universities don't have much to offer in this field. I had resigned myself to study something else, but now my dream will be fulfilled, thanks to you both!" There was no sense denying it, I felt that our effort had been well rewarded by our son's words and excitement.

Immediately John Paul wrote to various colleges in California and was accepted by the Glendale College in Pasadena. Our son left for Los Angeles January 8, 1980; he had just turned 19. His father traveled with him and rented a small furnished apartment not too far from the college. He opened a bank account in both their names for the periodical deposits we would send to cover the expenses. In no time J. P. adjusted well to his new habitat.

As for me I survived. Other than five months down the road, unable to resist the urge to see my son, I went to visit him. I arrived on a Friday and John Paul notified of my coming, the minute I got to the disembarking gate, jumped out from the crowd and came to greet me. I was lifted up from the floor in a powerful embrace. He was close to 6 feet, I only 5; 2, and in his arms, I swung around as if on a merry-go-round.

On the way out of the airport, chatting and laughing I found he had hired a limousine to drive us to his apartment; along the way, I enjoyed a couple of *Cuba Libres*, my favorite drink. John Paul had extended himself splendidly to give me a special welcome.

As I started to unpack my carry-on suitcase (my stay was only for four days), John Paul's friends began to show up to meet me. I saw a great conviviality among them and my son. Assured that he had not struggled with lonesomeness, I was glad.

For the weekend John Paul and his friends had interesting things programmed on my behalf, from Disneyland, to bars and nightclubs, and of course I paid. I noticed that one out of the bunch was like his shadow; where ever he went, Caroline was there too. She seemed madly in love with my son. I don't think he felt the same way for her, but J.P had no problem being worshiped by her.

What's more the girl had a car, and seemingly she had designated herself as his driver and during my stay, mine too She seemed to be a year or two older than J.P., blond, a bit heavier around the hips, the same height as my son and somewhat attractive, but not a beauty. I liked the girl anyway. I had the feeling John Paul would be well looked after by her.

On Monday I also had the chance to meet two of J. P.'s teachers, Tony his drawing instructor and Wayne, his teacher in sculpture. They were young and according to J.P. very skillful. Evidently they also appreciated him and his art too, a fact that made me extremely proud. Overall everything appeared okay. John Paul was a good student, excelling in art and I if at times saw marijuana joints crop up, didn't bother me. I knew my son's priorities were his studies. Satisfied, I returned home.

Once John Paul had successfully completed the two required semesters at in College, he was accepted in the University of Southern California, the same one where his Dad had graduated as a Petroleum Engineer. It was certainly more costly and it also demanded a high point average from John Paul's college accomplishments. Our son was very proud of this achievement.

We certainly lived well, perhaps a little on the flamboyant side; therefore we hardly had any savings. J. P.'s University, Patrick's school, a private one at that, the country club and the cars, the maid and the dogs. John and Patrick often visited John Paul, the same as myself, but we went separately because of our work and our younger son's schooling, besides that we also made sure J.P came home on summer and Christmas breaks; all took a fair chunk of the money we made. In addition my husband's other investments chiseled at it too but it didn't matter, we knew the source was unlimited; or at least we thought it was, as it kept on pouring in every month.

The country's financial system held strong even after the self-appointed dictator who had ruled the country for over a decade was forced to withdraw from political office in order to democratize the Nation. He ran as a candidate himself in the elections soon to be called.

Everything seemed in order and nothing perturbed our horizons until in the later part of September 1982, John, who was a healthy person, had an urological incident. Dr. Fernando Alvarez one of the best urologists in town as well as a good friend, performed an exploratory procedure and discovered a growth in John's bladder; a biopsy proved it was a malignant growth.

Panic-stricken I told my husband, "Honey, this is very serious. You need to go to the United States. The growth should be removed and treated over there. I'm sure the doctors in the States can work wonders. Isn't that so, I asked Fernando?"

Our friend, taking control of the situation, without dubitation answered, "Myriam if the surgical procedure is performed in the States it will cost you an arm and a leg, close to forty thousand dollars if not more considering plane tickets and recovery time." He then looking to my husband added, "I'm an experienced urologist; you know this John. I can do the operation myself. You just have to trust me."

"Will you be more specific Fernando," my husband asked, intrigued by our friend's words. "I'm well-prepared to perform the operation myself; in addition we have a good hospital here. If you accept my suggestion John, the cost will be entirely covered by your health insurance plan, but if you choose to go north, every cent will have to come out from your pocket," our friend answered.

Even with our two businesses flourishing nicely, we didn't have that kind of money on hand. My husband and I had to consider Fernando's opinion thoroughly before deciding to jump onto a plane. This time it was me who asked our friend to give us more details, which he did and completed his statement saying, "If after the operation I find anything abnormal, which I don't expect, I'll tell you immediately. At that point I will be the first to recommend the trip to the United States." His response satisfied us and John opted to stay.

Still it was difficult not to worry; we knew the consequences of malignancies, John and I had lost both our fathers to cancer, yet we tried to remain optimistic and shared our concern with our partner and his wife. Encouragingly they both gave us the support we needed; including financial backing from the factory in the eventuality John had to go to the States.

We didn't see the point in notifying John Paul. Apprehensive about his Dad, he would only drop his studies and return home. The gravity of John's health challenge was yet unknown, so we chose to tell our son everything after the surgery which because of the urgency took place only four days later.

Coming out from the operating room, still wearing his surgeon gown, Fernando with a great big smile on his face told me, "Everything went better than I expected, Myriam. We caught the growth at an early stage. It hadn't spread; it only penetrated two of the superficial layers. John's bladder is intact; I didn't have to remove it. He is going to be all right!" I could not have been more relieved. The frenzied life style we led hadn't compromised my love for John; no, it was just as strong as ever.

The likelihood that I might loose him had been eliminated. Yet like a doubting Thomas, I had to ask my friend, "Fernando, is he really going to be alright? You aren't just telling me this to appease my mind, are you?" "No Myriam I'm telling you the truth. The prognosis is even better than what I had anticipated; he should have periodic checkups but that is it. He doesn't need to go to the States, but if it will give you both peace of mind, John is free to go. I'll prepare all the necessary reports to help out." Believing him now, I gave Fernando a huge hug and thanked for all he had done.

With that weight lifted off of my shoulders, the minute I got home I called John Paul. He more or less accepted my explanation, but skeptical said, "Mom, I know Doctor Alvarez is good, but I'm not too sure about the hospital; I don't think it has all the modern technology we have here in California. To be on the safe side, I will make an appointment with a specialist in Los Angeles. I'll call you back the moment I have the date. In the mean time give my love to Dad and take good care of him, okay?"

Fully recovered two months later John traveled to the United States. After a five thousand dollar consultation involving the clinic and the specialist, the American doctor confirmed the diagnosis and suggested the same as our friend; periodic check-ups every six months to ascertain the malignancy didn't recur. Was my husband cancer free? We didn't know, we only hoped.

Afterwards, the soirées entertaining clients or friends and of course the drinking the whole old routine was back. In the midst of this *fandango* a prominent general in the army through some mutual friends had expressed his interest in buying our house. He knew our home was not on the market, but apparently the general had an interesting philosophy, "If the price is right everything is for sale." To some extent he was correct; his viewpoint coincided with mine.

A while back I had made my husband aware of my new aspirations, "Dear, I have been thinking that it would be a good idea if we sell our house. It's a beautiful home. I'm sure we can get an excellent price; with the money we can build a better one yet." I said it more than asked. John laughed at my suggestion. Probably he thought I was joking, but he then saw I was serious and said, "If its your dream dear, I'll go along with whatever makes you happy."

In recent years John and I had become party animals. We just plain liked to entertain! Bankers or prospective clients happened to be our most assiduous guests, but our friends also took part in our revelries. This was when I figured we needed some kind of a Hollywood style home to entertain even more; our two sons aware of my fantasies got excited and approved of my idea.

At forty-five I was still an attractive woman, plus intelligent; my husband, a born chevalier, was the first to always compliment my looks and my smarts. But as the arrogant fool I was becoming, I didn't see where I was heading. To be the heart of a party was my new image; to spark some jealousy in my female friends when I was invited to take part in civic or political events and they were not, gave me a secret joy. The success I was having in the business world apparently was going up to my head.

Ironically, it troubled me to take an initiative in matters of importance without our partner's consent. So I had to ask him,

"Mauricio, a Minister in the political arena wants to buy my house," I announced smiling teasingly, but looking for his approval.

"What! Your house is not for sale. Are you crazy?" he snapped in disbelief. "No, I'm serious. I'm actually dead serious on the money. Besides, you know we can always build another one, *si?*" Mauricio not happy with the way the conversation was going chose to ignore the subject hoping it would go away.

Not I, because the next time the Minister came to town, now aware that I was open to the idea, he approached us, "Myriam, John I understand you have a beautiful home, I would like to see it. I want to buy it for my wife. She would like to spend more time in Cochabamba; her mother lives here."

"If the price is right we certainly would consider it," I responded raising my hands and moving my fingers, pretending to count while at the same time we walked him through the house. He immediately fell in love with our place. We bargained a little, but in the end he accepted my price, an excellent one at that.

John didn't know that Mauricio was not too keen on the idea; the existing rivalry was just between our partner and myself. Of late I even sensed certain amount of jealousy in our partner's mindset, more so when he addressed specific subjects, such as when he questioned, "How is it that you guys have more than I have? You go on trips, while my family doesn't. I'm the creator of the industries and the general manager, I should have the same or more?"

"Undoubtedly you are all that Mauricio, but you also need to realize that John through his work earns an excellent salary and that I also work. In your case, you are the sole provider for your family; you have five offspring, while we only have two." I didn't know if my answer exasperated him even more or satisfied him, but the result was that he no longer addressed the subject.

Now it was time to give Mauricio my good news; that the sale was a done deal! I had the feeling he was not going to be too fascinated with my luck. Somehow I had to win him over. "The General has accepted to pay the amount I have asked for my house. Can you imagine all that we can do with that money? For a start, it would be great if we purchased the vacant lot next to our present house. It hasn't sold yet; I believe waiting for me to build another dream home, with your help of course. The owners are asking a fair price.

A big frowned appeared on his forehead and I heard some unintelligible noises coming out from his throat. But shortly after, composing himself in a clear voice Mauricio said, "Yes, certainly."

The general bought the house and in the interim we moved into one of the custom homes we'd previously built, unoccupied for the moment, but on the real estate market for sale. I had in mind to use the money from the sale only to my advantage, but my strategy didn't work as planed.

We purchased the lot next door and a few months down the road despite the fact that the entire concrete structure was completed and roofed, the hole in the ground for the swimming pool dug out; the completion of this magnificent home two and a half stories tall hung in the air. More pressing matters such as paying factory loans and other debts delayed the finishing.

It appeared that while I planned and dreamt, my countrymen who were not ready for democracy precipitated the downfall of the Bolivian economy!

DECEMBER 29, 1985

UNDETECTED, THE COCAINE HAD GONE THROUGH ALL INTERNAtional airports, including Paris. In Nice, where the plane had just landed, our luggage was not even searched. The finish line was in sight, I had nothing to fear anymore. Once I had settled with Judith, I planned to take a plane to Spain, deliver the drug, be paid for my troubles, and be on my way to see Luis José to collect the reference letter for the specialist in Paris.

While we waited for our luggage, I excused myself from my son, "Honey I have to go to the washroom, I'll be right back." Instead, I went to find a phone booth to make a call. Bernard's instructions had been very clear, "For safety, call Mario from a public telephone to set the time and place for the rendezvous in Barcelona."

This seemed the best chance I had; tapping my feet impatiently on the floor I muttered, "Hurry up Mario, answer the phone, I don't have much time." On the fourth ring, he did. Identifying myself, and smiling I said, "I'm here in Nice, Mario. All went well. When do we meet?"

"That's great; I've been expecting your call. How does this Thursday sound? I'll meet you at three o'clock at the Buena Vista Motel in Barcelona. The motel is located at the corner of Calle 94 and Figueroa. You can't miss it. I'll wait for you in the lobby."

I agreed, and the click of the receiver being hung up at the other end came as a happy hum in my ears. Everything had gone as planned, only two more days and my son and I would be flying back to Paris, to see the specialist! As I returned to John Paul's side, I saw he had our suitcases and was ready to go. We walked to the main gate, where Judith agreed to wait for us.

The minute I saw her all I wanted was to ask her, "Have you completed the deal? Is the cocaine sold, and do you have the money?" The fact that I was now in Nice with the extra 700 grams was only because of her inaptitude. Judith had put me through a lot trouble, but because J. P. was with me, I held back.

Judith must have sensed I was not in a good mood, and acting as a gracious host, perhaps to ease the atmosphere she said, "To go to my house, which is located in a small hill in Mandelieu-Cannes, I will take you through the scenic route bordering the Mediterranean Sea." Showing indifference I just nodded. As Judith began the drive, a tourist spill started, "We are driving through *Le Promenade des Anglais;* Nice's main boulevard well known for the classy hotels and villas facing the ocean."

It was true. Stunning buildings stood at one side of the avenue; it was all fascinating and of course I couldn't help being keyed up admiring the splendor, while John Paul just quietly sat in the back seat watching my excitement. J.P. had traveled these roads before when he first visited France.

Judith then changing the subject jubilantly shared her good news, "Jean Pierre is home now. He has returned from Africa; he'll be spending Christmas plus some extra time with me and the kids." "You must be thrilled. I understand it was difficult for him to take time off from work during the holiday season. You had a nice surprise didn't you? Now we'll enjoy him too!" I said sarcastically but happy for her.

As we continued the drive, Judith pointed out to the Ste. Marguerite Ile, supposedly the island where the Iron Mask man was imprisoned; some other islands, castles and for a while the scenery transported me back in time. I forgot everything.

It was just me, in one of Alejandro Dumas novels, *El Conde de MonteCristo*, or in *Los Tres Mosqueteros*, or perhaps in *El hombre de la Mascara de Hierro*.

As a child, later as a youth and much later as an adult, I loved to read novels, and biographies, and anything that had to do with world history. My father's excellent library nurtured my imagination which now ran wild because I was stepping on the soil in which some of those events took place.

The old monasteries and villas I saw at a distance held grand chronicles, first when the Royalty was prevalent, later with the French Revolution: altogether dramatic times. The magic I was submerged in was broken by Judith's next words pointing out something else, "We are now driving through the *Boulevard de la Croisette*, entering Cannes."

Again, to my right I had the breathtaking sight of the *Cote d'Azure* and to my left impressive buildings; no wonder the rich and famous loved to vacation around this area. As the road started up hill, Judith completed our tour saying, "We are approaching my house. You have to see the view we have; it's beautiful." She was right again; they had a gorgeous view of the city.

As soon as we arrived, Jean Pierre and their two children came out to meet us and helped with our luggage. I had met Jean Pierre before when they both came to visit Judith's father and extended their visit to us. He received us courteously, had some hors d'oeuvres and drinks ready to share with us. I felt good! In this easygoing atmosphere, with soft music playing in the background, my stress vanished. I even enjoyed the *pisco sours* Jean Pierre prepared for us and relaxed some more. Dinner came a little later.

We had traveled for more than thirty-two hours straight to meet connecting flights; John Paul, exhausted, found his own way to the guest quarters and retired for the night. It was the opportune moment to talk in private to Judith, so excusing myself to Jean Pierre I asked her, "Judith will you show me the way to my quarters?"

Once alone I peppered her with my questions, "Did your friend sell the cocaine? Do you have the money now?" Hesitantly and with a slight tremor on her lower lip she responded, "No. Everything has been postponed." Dumbfounded by her answer, I felt my temper rising, ready to explode. I had warned her that I didn't want to hear any more excuses or delays and now she was telling me different.

Somehow I managed to keep my anger under control and allowed Judith to continue explaining, "The buyer wants to deal directly with you. He is interested in buying the portion you brought as well." Judith, with an obvious naiveté had relayed to her friend everything I told her in our last telephone conversation, "I've purchased more cocaine which I intend to sell myself; I've got to make up for my losses. I have a more reliable contact elsewhere."

All was correct, but Judith should have kept the information to herself. Now to justify this new stupid delay, she blabbered some more, "As soon as my friend's contact learned you were bringing more cocaine, he wanted to wait and talk to you personally. He thought he could persuade you to negotiate the sale of the whole amount with him instead." I could not have been more annoyed; in my view the entire affair with her friend and the contact was a total fiasco. I didn't want to continue with it; I had an uneasy feeling about the whole deal.

Furious with Judith's excuses, I impatiently told her, "I really don't trust your friend and her people anymore. I've wasted far too much time as it is. You had your chance, I've already arranged things with someone dependable in Spain; it's where I intend to go shortly. I'm sure he'll even buy the part you brought. I would much rather deal with him now."

Judith, who failed to see my point stubbornly argued, "I don't agree with you. I happen to know my friend very well too, and she is trustworthy; I can't go back on my word now. You have to understand my side as well." Here we were, arguing like two small children in such a serious matter, but after all what did we know about what we were in, we were only amateurs.

Convinced by her words I decided to compromise, "Okay, I will let you keep the seven hundred grams you brought. You can complete the deal with your friend's contact, but that's it. I don't want to hear of any more delays!" Too tired from the long voyage, I didn't tell Judith that my trip to Spain was scheduled for Thursday; it was now Tuesday past midnight. *We have talked enough; I can always tell her tomorrow*, I told myself, as I wished her good night.

J.P. was sound asleep. Quietly I went to bed and even though I had stopped interacting with God long ago; I was certain that it was Him who had protected me in my journey. I now found it quite natural to thank Him for his help.

A little while later I was also asleep. I have no idea for how long I had been in Morpheus' arms when suddenly I was awakened. Judith was standing by my bed talking to me. At first, nothing she said made any sense, but as I woke up, her words became clearer but there was no rhyme or reason to what she was saying.

"A few minutes ago two men came; they were looking for you. I don't understand why my friend didn't advise me they were coming tonight. Not prepared for this intrusion, afraid the noise would wake up my husband, I told them you were not here. I sent them away but not before I agreed you would meet with them at the Mall's parking lot, Thursday at 11:00 am.

Fully awake now, I looked at my watch and snapped back, "That is the day after tomorrow. I can't meet with those men; I'll be in Spain by then. Actually I'll be leaving on the first available plane!" Judith, indignant because I hadn't told her my trip to Spain was that soon, grumbled, "What do you expect me to do now? The rendezvous is already arranged."

I wasn't happy either. She hadn't consulted with me about the last dealings she made with her friend. So in no mood to listen any more, I told her, "You'll have to be the one to meet with those men. That is if you still want to deal with them. After all they're your friend's contacts, not mine. Unless you'd rather I take the problem off your hands. You decide." Judith agreed to deliver the stuff herself.

After she left the room I could not sleep anymore, I was still dealing with her intrusion but more pressing stuff crammed my brain. In close proximity to my objective, the money from Spain and consequently John Paul's treatment, I didn't need any other kind of interferences.

Early in the morning I called several travel agencies to book my flight to Barcelona, but it proved to be futile, the New Year was approaching and all flights were sold out. An unexpected obstacle that forced me to alter my plans; I would rent a car and drive to Barcelona instead.

With this settled in my mind, I accepted Judith's invitation to spend the rest of the day sightseeing Cannes, our discussion of the night over and done. The tour turned out impressive, since I had the chance to check the celebrated Hotel Martinez and some other beautiful buildings and places. Later in the day Jean Pierre and the children joined us and we dined at a grilled and wine restaurant in town. I treated, I would not have it otherwise, not after the great hospitality displayed by them. Because of the children, the evening ended fairly early

When John Paul and I were alone, I deceivingly told him, "I just learned my friend Luis José is going in holidays tomorrow and unfortunately all the flights to Barcelona are booked solid. I need to be there tomorrow, no later than three o'clock in the afternoon to collect the letter; otherwise we will miss the chance to get it. I will rent a car; would you drive me there? You know how much I hate long-distance driving."

It was another lie, as the doctor was not going anywhere. He actually was going to wait for me. It was me who needed to be there on time to close my business deal. Once in Barcelona, my plan was to find a motel where we would stay overnight, leave my son settled there, and then continued in a taxi to the Buena Vista Motel, deliver the drug, and be paid.

Once the deal was concluded, on my way back get the referral letter from Luis José and I could easily return to my son's side with the money and the letter by five. All fit perfectly well, more so when my son, only too happy to be of some help said, "I'd love to go with you to Spain, Mom." Strangely that night I didn't toss or twist on my bed thinking of the steps I was to take the next day; I slept like a baby, as if I had no worries in the world.

Clear-headed and well dressed the next morning I asked Judith. "Could you please drop us off at a car-rental. I need to rent a car to go to Spain?"

"Of course Myriam no problem," she responded and immediately we loaded our suitcases in her car, the cocaine still in mine. At the automobile location, I paid cash for the lease, but for security reasons the clerk requested my surrogate cousin to endorse the agreement. With everything in place, we said good-bye to Judith and headed for Barcelona.

Unsuspicious of anything, John Paul at the wheel said, "We'll be there by two o'clock." It was seven now. Carefree, sure all the dangers were behind, I could almost taste the victory. Had I not gone through the most difficult places undetected? The crossing of the French and Spanish border shouldn't pose a concern.

After Barcelona we were going to Paris, and John Paul surely would start with the treatment. None of the symptoms were back, the fever, the swelling of lymph's nodes, or the other stuff, everything seemed to be normal for the moment, which allowed me to think that if JP's condition had been stationary, the more chance he had to be cured. In this frame of mind, I fully enjoyed the scenery of southern France.

My son, undoubtedly a good driver, controlled the car well. The highway often seemed as though it would merge into the Mediterranean, an unparallelled special effect.

Though it was winter and a strong wind blew from east to west, the scenery of the Cote d'Azure was undoubtedly breathtaking. We could imagine its magnificence in summer and pondered the life of the rich and famous as we drove past many luxurious hotels and resorts. Jokingly we even envisioned vacationing here and sailing on our own private yacht. No harm in dreaming!

The cities of Aix-en-Provence, Marseilles, Nimes, Montpellier, Beziers went by. It was almost two o'clock in the afternoon; our butts a little stiff from the long drive looked forward to a stretch out in Perpignan, the border town. About five kilometers from the town, John Paul directed my attention to the many police cars that were in the vicinity, seemingly approaching the gates of the border simultaneously with us.

Only after John Paul had mentioned it, I noticed the vehicles. Unconcerned I made a couple of smart remarks about them. "I wonder what high ranking politician is expected for such a patrol? Or maybe it is destined for important people like us?" I laughed, making a joke out of the situation.

Our turn came to present our passports. The customs officer who took them confirmed our identities addressing us by our names, Mrs. Myriam Arthur, Mr. John Paul Arthur, while at the same time glancing at the pictures on the documents.

We didn't get them back. Suddenly the cruisers no longer at a distance encircled us. Similar to what I had seen in the big screen, where the police cordoned gangsters in a delinquent activity. It was unreal, and not a few minutes earlier, I had even joked with my son about the platoon, never imagining that those police vehicles could actually be a welcoming committee for me!.

It had to be a mistake; I was no mobster!

PART II

December 31, 1985

Still in the car, John Paul turning his head towards me and with his beautiful hazel-green eyes sadden said, Mom I had the feeling something was wrong as far back as our initial flight to France, but I stopped my questioning after you assured me that everything was okay. I chose to ignore the voice within trying to get my attention.

We had no chance to talk anymore. Heavily escorted my son and I were directed inside the building and placed in two separate rooms; our suitcases fetched from the trunk were left in the front room.

My heart pounded so hard it felt as if it was going to come out from my chest; my head ached as if someone was hammering inside and I felt as though the world be caving in on me. Somehow I managed to control my panic and forced myself to investigate my surroundings. From the small window in the room I was able to peek into an adjacent area, which seemed to be a garage and I saw that my rental car was being stripped; off the seats went, the inside door covers too. Next, the tires were dismounted and every detachable piece was meticulous removed and inspected.

In total denial, I fancied the search was performed only because the car had to be a stolen vehicle, used by someone else in other illegal activity, nothing to do with me! In my view, the out-and-out hunt could only be related to Mafia dealings; why, otherwise the incredible display of police force? It had to be directed to the head of a big *Mafioso* gang?

After the long search and the car totally stripped, the French officers had nothing to show from their rummaging around, the heads shaking and loud utterances proved their frustration. My anxiety escalated. Was their hunt after all for the cocaine? Someone must have alerted the authorities; I wondered who?

I retraced my steps carefully. I went as far back as when I contacted the boys and asked for their help; and listened to Bernard's words of advice, "The success of your venture depends in how well you wrap the cocaine. People are caught if isn't well done. The battle won't be over until all customs are behind you, the drug delivered and the payment claimed."

Thanks to the warning, I hit on the unique packaging for the drug; method that proved safe when Judith took the cocaine, as well as for me to this point. Undetected, the drug had gone through various airports; if Customs and Immigration officials were suspicious, they would have captured me on the spot, not waited this long to make an arrest.

Bernard went even further in his advise, "In all pre-arranged meetings, you need to be punctual. If one is delayed, no phone calls are advisable and the wait shouldn't exceed more than one hour. Automatically it would be assumed something had gone wrong and each should look out for their safety." From the beginning all he wanted to do was protect me. Why would he go to that extreme if he planned to give me away?

It couldn't be Bernard who alerted the authorities. What if my connection in Barcelona had turned sour? I ruled out this possibility too, it was a link Bernard had given me. Besides, if Mario wanted to double-cross me he would have waited until I was in Spain, otherwise what would be his gain? In Cochabamba, the only one who knew of my activity was Rose. She was too close a friend to betray my trust.

Bit by bit I went over these details, still unable to figure out how the information could have leaked. Furthermore, no one knew I would be going to Spain by car, not until the day before when unexpected circumstances made me changed the plan on my itinerary! It had to be that something had wrong in Cannes. Judith was the only one who knew where I was going. Could she have been the one to inform the police? Hard to believe, yet everything pointed to her.

A group of officers entering the room interrupted my reflections. Their icy stare gave me the chills. Frightened I didn't dare move or say anything. In broken English, one of them said, "Hand over your purse." It was still in my hands. I obeyed.

Then a uniformed woman motioned to follow her, opened a door leading to a bathroom. I didn't know what to expect. She articulated some words in French. Seeing I didn't understand, she signaled me to take off my clothes, including my brassier and underwear. In the nude, I stood for what it seemed an eternity, while she examined me the clothes piece-by-piece. Whatever the woman was searching for, the result was negative as she found nothing.

She then silently put on a pair of surgical gloves and gestured me to bend from the waist down frontward, my derriere facing her. This could only mean she intended to perform a body cavity search. I gasped for air and trembled. My humiliation was so great that I broke into tears.

Did the women feel sorry for me? Likely yes, because suddenly she didn't continue with the task; instead she motioned me to get dressed. I thanked God I was spared from such a horror. As we went back to the other room, foolishly I asked the one who spoke English before, who seemed to act as some kind of interpreter, "Why are we detained?" His response came loud and abrupt, "The French authorities are aware of your trafficking. It'll make things easier on you if you cooperate with us." Nothing was found yet, so I didn't answer.

The officers then proceeded to open my son's suitcase; they carefully examined item-by-item and found nothing incriminating. My purse came next in their scrutiny, and the $800.00 American dollars I brought for our traveling expenses was retrieved, as well as my son's Bolivian passport and my own. Too worried about what they would find in my suitcase, the gestures and noises the Custom agents made as they put the items aside didn't draw my attention.

Now it was my bag being dissected. It seemed as if they were almost ready to give up on the search, when one of the Custom Agents touched the bottle of shampoo. He noticed its rigidity unusual for a container of shampoo. It was the cocaine stuffed to the rim.

He didn't open the bottle yet; first he called the attention of the other Customs officials. They exchanged a few words, and then all toiletries were separated and opened. In seconds he had in hands the second piece of evidence, the bottle of hair conditioner. Eureka! They all exploded, and got engaged in a loud and excited conversation!

While me, I wanted to die. I couldn't pretend anymore; frightened or not I had to do something, say something credible that will help me out. In my stupor, I came up with the naïve story that the suitcase was not mine that I was only delivering it for someone else

A pitiful scheme for an excuse, but I blabbered it anyway, "I was asked to deliver the suitcase to a man in Barcelona and get paid for my troubles. He is waiting for me at this address." Sure that by now my contact in Spain would not be waiting any longer and that his safety would not be compromised, I gave a fictitious name, but the right address. I thought if told part of the truth, it would be enough to satisfy their demand to collaborate.

But then there was my son; I had been so eager, better say stupid that I brought John Paul with me on such a dangerous expedition. He knew nothing about my plot, so urgently I needed to clarify the matter of his innocence too. John Paul had enough on his plate; my son shouldn't be mixed-up in my crime.

So I explained, "I'm not good at driving long distances. My son came along only because he is an experienced driver, but he didn't know I carried a suitcase that was not mine." I thought that this simple declaration from my part would clear my son.

Unable to see the reality that I faced, still in a mist, I remember seeing in motion pictures that following an arrest the suspect was read his rights and allowed to have a lawyer before any questioning even begin. In my capture none of this was happening.

Was it up to me to ask for legal counsel? Surely an attorney would set things straight. Armed with a new courage, I demanded in Spanish, "*Necesito ver un abogado.*" No response. I wondered if these people didn't understand Spanish, so I repeated my request in English, "I need to see a lawyer" I got the same blank look in their faces. Yet, the one who seem to act as interpreter said something that sounded English, "We are *Douane* Agents, we have no control over these matters. *Vous doit presenter votre* demand to the Police Detectives, due to come soon." And that was the end of it.

The wait was infernally long. My mind wondered back and forth as to what I should do or not. Finally two men dressed in civilian clothes showed up; apparently the investigators. My son, who all this time had been detained in another room, rejoined me; he was handcuffed, I was not. Seeing my son treated in such a manner felt as if someone was piercing my heart with a dagger. He had done nothing wrong and posed little threat to anyone.

Unexpectedly one of officers released him from the handcuffs. J.P. then came over and embraced me. "Will you be ever able to forgive me? You were right, I have done something terribly wrong," I said and began to cry. His embrace became more powerful as he spoke, "Mother, if anyone needs to be forgiven, it's me. Now I'm certain it's because of me you got into this mess. Please, Mom, don't cry. I'm sure everything will be all right." He reassured me, trying to appease my despair.

In the meantime the other policeman, who was being briefed on what happened, made it a point to harshly look over his shoulder whenever he faced us. He appeared hostile and his menacing front frightened me even more, as he came towards us. It made me wonder if this man was capable of torturing people in order to obtain the answers he expected.

"*Reprendrez-vous votres valises,*" the detective roughly said. The motion he made to pick up our suitcases helped to comprehend his command. We then tagged along behind him and his colleague out of the building and into their vehicle. The one who had un-cuffed my son, who seemed a kinder person, in broken English commented, "We are taking you to the police headquarters in Perpignan for further questioning." It was five in the afternoon, and the dark night had already set in.

The nasty one barked more unintelligible words, but seeing the futility of his effort added in English, "The French police are aware of your trafficking. Judith, who has been detained in Cannes, has confessed. I suggest you do the same." His words and demeanor could not be more boorish.

All became clear now; my childhood friend, my surrogate cousin, was the one who had given me away. Something definitely must have gone wrong at the rendez-vous and in a panic she told everything to the authorities; even my trip to Spain. She perhaps exposed me to save herself? The thought enraged me; Judith freely had chosen to go ahead with the deal. She ought not to have spilled anything. Enraged I wished her the worst.

It was impossible to maintain my first deposition now; no matter the consequences, the complete truth had to come out as soon as we got to the station. But my resolution had to wait longer because no sooner had we arrived than John Paul was the first to be taken into an adjacent chamber, where apparently the interrogation would take place. While guarded by two uniformed police officers I waited, seated on a bench next to the door that had just closed behind my son.

Minutes went by turning into one hour or maybe even more. Why the long interrogatory, I asked myself? He knows nothing about the situation. He only had to explain the circumstances surrounding the trip and the reason why he happened to be with me! Time stood still and my imagination went wild with the wait. I didn't know anything about French laws, or the language, but my knowledge of their history was extent. It led me to think he was locked in a dark dungeon, where I would soon be placed too.

Finally John Paul came out. He seemed intact; no harm had come to him. In spite of that the chance to talk to him faded away, as I was immediately ushered into the same room. No torturing tools in sight; just the two civilian officers, plus another man, whom was presented as the interpreter and a woman in front of a typewriter, but no signs of a lawyer.

Since Judith had succumbed, I had in mind to clarify my first statement but that was easier said than done. The translation into English complicated the issue. For the past 20 years I resided in Bolivia, a Spanish speaking country, and in the previous six years that I lived in North America, I never mastered the language. As a result English was still quite foreign for me, and didn't seem to be the interpreter's forté either; at least not in my ears. Yet no one had bothered to ask my preference for the language that should be used in the interpretation.

Thus, in a language I seldom used, I tried to explain, "The moment of my arrest I didn't tell the whole truth. I was too scared and confused. I'm still frightened, but I'm now ready to take full responsibility for my actions." In short I told everything, from beginning to end. I even broke my promise and revealed my son's illness; terrified more for him and his health than for myself, I released everything hoping to obtain some understanding.

The callous investigator did all the questioning translated for my benefit into English by the interpreter. As the inquest got rolling, the gaps between what the inept interpreter and I said were profound. More often than not, my answers had to be repeated several times, it went the same the other way around; surely a disadvantage for me.

"Give your full name." «Myriam Del Castillo de Arthur.»

"Where are you from?" "Cochabamba, Bolivia, South America."

"Are you married?" "Yes."

"Who is the man arrested with you?" "My son."

"Where is your husband?" "In Canada."

"Where do you live?" "In Bolivia."

"You both have two sets of passports, a Bolivian and a Canadian, certainly fraudulent and used for your trafficking purposes."

"No they are not. My son and I have dual citizenship. I'm Bolivian by birth and Canadian by marriage as a landed immigrant. My son is Canadian by birth and Bolivian by registration. We both reside in Bolivia and as Bolivian citizens we are compelled to display Bolivian documentation when leaving the country. Most countries required Bolivian passports to bear visas when entering their territory, a formality not needed by Canadian citizens. This is the reason why we travel with our two sets of passports!"

I had the feeling that not much of what I said was understood; for starters I didn't see the transcriber jot it down.

"You were under police surveillance. We know you and your son are involved in drug trafficking and are linked with a big ring of drug dealers. It's to your advantage to give a truthful statement. We want the names of every one involved with you here in France, as well as all of your other contacts."

Stupefied by the charges, though terrified, I maintained some presence of mind. It was impossible for the French police to know about my experimental trip to Brazil. Furthermore, to accuse me of being engaged with heavy duty mobsters, when never in my life had I previous association with the underworld, except for the three young man back home, who in my view had no leg on which to stand on as a ring of dealers. In addition to say that my son was involved, necessarily had to be false accusations only to frighten me. This convinced me that I should not be intimidated.

"There must be a mistake. I'm not a big trafficker. This is the first time I'm involved in something of this sort, in which my son had no part. As I said before, John Paul has AIDS and I resorted to trafficking because I needed the money to obtain medical attention for him. I don't work for anyone and I don't have anybody working for me, either."

Infuriated and in tears, I continued. "I've already admitted my guilt, but not in the manner you are implying. I bought the cocaine myself. On my way to deliver it and be paid, I was arrested. The custom agents at the border have this information, including the tentative meeting place where I was supposed to meet my contact in Barcelona and his name."

"From where do you know this man?" Bombarded with so many questions, this one unexpected, I candidly told the truth about how I happened to meet Jim, thinking it would help clear up matters.

"Long before my problem began, my husband and I learned an American young man was detained for possession of drugs at the city jail in my hometown. He had neither family nor friends, so as ambassadors of good will we brought food and some toiletries not provided by the prison system. Upon his release he married a Bolivian girl and remained in Cochabamba. I didn't see much of him after that. When my son got sick, I looked him up, hoping he could help me find a contact. He did help me; the contact was in Barcelona."

"What are their names?" I had stated a truthful fact but that was it. I was not about to get Jim, Bernard or Mario in trouble. After all, it was not them who had got me involved in trafficking; it was I who had requested their help. I could not double-cross them now, no matter how deeply in trouble I was. So I answered the question, giving false names, "The man in Barcelona's name is Mario Maldonado and as I said before, I don't even know him. The one in Bolivia, his name is Jim Barnett."

"From whom did you buy the cocaine and how much did you pay for it?" "I gave the money to Jim, to buy it for me. I paid ten thousand American dollars. I borrowed the money for the purchase."

"You don't seem to be hurting for money. You've traveled a lot, to Canada, United States, Argentina, Brazil, and Peru. Your passports bear stamps of your visits to those countries; you might even have more passports that we aren't aware off."

In no way could I explain the unrelated circumstances for those trips. It was a situation that now wrongly but clearly seemed to incriminate me. I realized the odds were against me! It would be very difficult to change the preconceived ideas these people were forming against me. Besides I was still sure my answers were not getting across.

"My family is well-known and respected in Bolivia. At one time we had the money to travel to those countries you mentioned, sometimes in leisure trips, others work related; we are part owners of a marble factory and a construction company. Adverse circumstances in my country caused a breakdown in the economy, money became scarce and then my son got ill. It would be easy for Interpol to verify my words. I want to make it very clear that my son had no part in my wrongdoing."

The officers continued with the questioning, but gave me the impression I was fighting a set idea, so I offered to undergo a polygraph test to prove I was not lying. It was not performed.

"What about Judith, who is also under arrest?" the tough guy asked. I had no clue to what could have gone wrong or the extent of her confession but I felt I needed to be cautious with this answer. My initial anger had subsided and I could not just point an accusing finger towards her involvement.

"Before Jim assisted me with a contact in Spain, I asked her to help me find a buyer for the cocaine here in France, but she was unable to execute my request. Subsequently, Jim found the counterpart in Spain."

My questioning seemed to have stopped. The two policemen began to talk to each other; the fear and anxiety I felt now, was comparable to the agony and pain I had when I first learned John

Paul was infected with AIDS, but compounded. I had not solved anything and here we were in this horrible predicament instead.

Shortly after the interpreter said, "You and your son will remain detained in Perpignan; a judge will decide whether your case will be transferred to Nice or sustained under this jurisdiction." Our arrest happened in the vicinity of Perpignan, while Judith's took place in Nice, apparently the reason.

The gravity of my situation sank deeper, but despite everything, the thought of imprisonment was far from my mind. I was convinced that once the procedures were filled, the judge, aware of my circumstances would understand. I would be severely reprimanded, but not incarcerated and John Paul's innocence would not even be questioned.

I was certainly reinventing the law, assuming that my assertion of guilt was all that was needed for the release of my son. What I didn't realize was that under French law, offenders when arrested didn't have any rights; the drug was found in my possession, thus I was considered a criminal and in a domino effect my son's innocence and credibility was also at stake, because he happened to be with me. In any event, I was sure a lawyer would set the matter straight, but my request to see one was ignored.

Led back to where John Paul sat, I saw he had been handcuffed again; ashamed, I didn't dare look at my son. Yet I knew he deserved an explanation. Holding back my tears, with quavering voice I told him, "John Paul, I've deceived you, your father and everyone else, about promoting an export business trip to France, all nothing but a lie! When in reality it is cocaine that I brought, to sell to pay for the medical help you needed, but look what I have caused instead? I should have never have brought you with me!"

My confession out in the open, I was unable to contain the flow of tears. Seeing my anguish, John Paul didn't confront me, or accuse me, on the contrary he only comforted me, "Please Mother, don't cry. Everything will be all right, I am sure." Our intimate moment was cut short when the two investigators ordered us to follow them.

Guided by them we marched into another area, but in the same building. Here my son and I were photographed and fingerprinted; all seemed more like a figment of my imagination and it was not over yet. The march continued further, inside the precinct where John Paul and I were placed behind bars in two separate cells.

As I entered the one assigned to me, the stench of some repulsive stuff on the floor beside the narrow bench where I was supposed to rest my weary body, hit me. It seemed to be vomit and blood. The repugnant sight, plus the appalling experience from before was just too much. I closed my eyes and I must have blacked out.

The sound of laughter and the background blare, plus the rattling of my teeth from the chill of the night brought me back to my present and brutal reality. I was in jail somewhere in France! I still wore my elegant winter coat; it was good for mild winters but gave me no protection from the cell's dampness. I felt as if I had been tossed into a deep freezer. Concerned I tried to recall if John Paul was wearing something warm.

I looked around and found that all the noise came from an oval room, where men in uniform, likely in charge of the precinct, were having some kind of a celebration. My watch read ten o'clock; seven hours since the moment we were stopped at the border; perhaps only minutes in the cell, yet to me it felt like an eternity.

Additional officers arrived over crowding the oval space; their voices and laughter grew louder while consuming a red beverage, likely wine. Nothing more out of place, police officers drinking on the job! My thoughts reverted to the nasty stuff I seen next to the bench. No matter how hard I tried to keep my eyes away from the mess, my gaze was glued to the sight.

In my mind's eyes, I saw the same police officers pulverizing a defenseless person, one blow after another on the stomach and face until he bled and vomited, perhaps to death. I got more scared. What could I expect from them now that the alcohol seemed to be going to their heads? But I stopped and didn't allow my brain to go any further. I forced myself to ignore what I just seen or imagined?

A break in the noise brought my attention to a whispering voice from the adjoining cell. It was John Paul's and he was calling me, "Mom, Mom are you okay? I hope you aren't crying. I'm fine, just tired and there is another young man in my cell. I haven' t had chance to speak with him yet, because he is sleeping. You won't believe this; he's sleeping on the floor covered with just a blanket. I'm beat Mom. I think I'll do the same." John Paul said yawning. "Call me if you are afraid, you know I'm near you. Yes Mom, I do have a warm jacket and Mom will you try to get some rest too. Okay?"

My son's comforting words lifted the terror in which I had surrounded myself. The jail cell was still the same, dirty, damp and probably the darkest place I have ever been. But the difference now was that my son's voice broke the sinister spell I had wrapped myself in. It helped me think on higher notes and concentrate on a way I could obtain contact with my husband.

John had to know everything, and I realized that it was not going to be easy to explain the hell of a mess I had made. Worse yet admit my blunder, John Paul should not ever have come to France with me; not while the cocaine was in my possession anyway, even if my intent appeared to have had a good purpose. I had risked his safety and we were now both in a jail, with no lawyer in sight and no access to doctors!

In a roller-coaster of emotions, a refusal to accept the gravity of my offense took over again, and I saw myself as a champion, instead of an offender. Consequently punishment was out of the question, perhaps deported but nothing else. Continuing in the same foolishness, I even thought that once the judge learned of our situation John Paul would be checked by a doctor, even treated and once at home, no one other than John and maybe Mauricio would know of my mishap.

The cheering helped me for an instant, but the fact that at one point I would need to confront John and our partner with the truth frighten me. I didn't know how on earth would I be able to do it? Fearless I had gone on about my mission, but I now lacked courage to face the music my action had created. What could I possibly say to my husband anyway?

Explain things that were impossible to justify? No matter what I said, or how I put it, John surely will despise me. What about Patrick, what would our younger son think? Would he be able to understand that in my eagerness to help his brother, knowingly I took a detour to the wrong? I now wished that in his young heart, Patrick would only see the good side of my objective.

Then there was my mother. All she knew was that I went to Brazil on a business trip; finding out that I was jailed in France instead could easily kill her. Mom had some heart problems, now I feared for her health. My intent backfired and not only had I not resolved anything about our crisis; on the contrary all I accomplished was to intensify the problem.

Only at this point did I realize the pathetic absurdities of my measures. Why didn't I consider the consequences of my actions before? Why did I ignore the likelihood that something like this could happen, even if the warnings came very frailly, why?

Evidently because I felt my mission was protected; to the point that even now I failed to grasp the seriousness of my offense. I appreciated it as a disgraceful act but that was it, my circumstances had prompted me to proceed and I still held firm to the belief that with the help of a lawyer my situation would be cleared.

December 31, 1985

In spite of my comforting thoughts, the reality of the surroundings was overpowering. The blast in the oval room had increased; the officers now sang and danced, embraced and kissed each other, while I didn't even dare move. I didn't want to attract unwanted attention. No idea what was taking place, but soon it dawned on me, it was New Year's Eve!

The more they celebrated the New Year the more beaten I felt by the misery of our status. "Mom, Mom." Once again my son's voice came in my rescue. "Mom, come to the front of your cell, I want to try something. Maybe I can hold your hand."

Momentarily I put my somber thoughts aside, replaced by the eagerness to do exactly as I was told. I twisted my body side ways and en-twisted the other way, stretching my left arm through the bars as far out as possible. While John Paul's grunting proved he was doing the same in a backbreaking effort, but in the end we were only able to touch the tips of our fingers. Not much, but it certainly gave me a jolt of good energy.

Next John Paul said, "Happy New Year, Mom! Please don't worry so much, okay? God knows you are the kindest person in the world. He also knows if you made this mistake, it was only because you wanted to help me."

I tried to say something, but it was my son who continued, talking, "So, you see, Mom, I'm just as guilty and I believe I know what the Lord wants from me. He wants me to be near you, to give you my love and support through this crisis, the same as you always have done for me. Cheer up Mom; soon we'll be both out of here. Now try to get some rest, okay?" My son's comforting words made me feel undeservedly blessed.

Later the frigidity of the cell and lack of movement got me shivering. My legs were numb, my bones ached and even my bladder began to give me trouble. When I first came into the cell, I had I looked with disgust the two dirty blankets folded at the foot of the bench. Now hoping I would warm up a bit, reluctantly I reached for the least dirty to cover my legs.

Intimidated, without other woman in the precinct, I wanted to pass unseen at least until daybreak. Except that my bladder didn't agree with my wishes and I was forced to notify my discomfort to someone. A guard approached the cell and after he learned of my need, the officer opened the barred door and escorted by him I was lead to the washroom through a dark and narrow hallway.

The moment I walked in, I wished I didn't have to use it! The ancient toilette bowl that at one time must have been white now was brown! The smell made my stomach turn. Not to mention the cockroaches that ran into hiding the moment the light switch was turned on. Even so, nature was stronger than what my eyes and nose couldn't stand; it just took its course.

On the way back, I noticed John Paul trying to get the guard's attention. He too wanted to go to the bathroom. I had the feeling it was more of an excuse to ensure my safety with his presence, even if his situation wasn't any better. To have my son watching over me was a great comfort, and again helped calm my nerves.

More conscious after the short walk, I realized my daydreaming had to stop. My mess would never be solved on its own. No matter how much I dreaded the thought, John had to be notified; he had to learn where we were. Once he was aware of the seriousness of our son's health, of our situation, I was sure my husband would do anything in his power to assist his son and who knows even help me.

John loved John Paul just as much as I did. He would not hesitate in sacrificing everything we owned, if it meant helping either one of our sons. Deep down in heart, I knew that I could have done the same, but instead I closed my eyes and opted out for an erroneous road. Only now in the solitude of my own thoughts, I decided to unearth my sole and find what I had done wrong or failed to do that so drastically made me detour from the good road. I knew I could not change a thing, but I had to know?

It was true that after my father's death my character changed. I became more detached because along the way on the face of it, I lost the zealous faith I once had for the Lord. Then as we succeeded in business, without His backing, my ego gained terrain and my cynicism grew in unparalleled measures. It was easy for me to find the smallest of faults in everyone around me, even in good solid people, while I exempted myself from having any.

We had busy lives alright, John traveled constantly with his consulting job, while I helped Mauricio manage both our business and I didn't notice that I was more interested in climbing the corporate world than to keep our house in order.

Wrapped up in this frivolous behavior, subtlety the changes had crept in me, so insignificant at first that I didn't noticed. Except that I believe God knew, but kept a silent watch over me and I failed the test. Slowly and without much effort my new way took over and all hell broke loose when John Paul came home and told me he was infected with AIDS. No need to deny it, I had triggered our present situation myself.

I just couldn't stop thinking about what I had done and while doing so it allowed me to discover other unpleasant facts about myself. Baffled by pain, under subterfuges I brought my son to France in search of medical help and accomplished the opposite. True that we didn't have cash on hand and again true that the banks would not lend money, not even in American dollars; but I believe the embryo of greed played a major part in preventing me from talking about our financial crisis with my husband.

John would have insisted on selling our assets. I knew the option was there, but following the country's economic collapse, the price of those assets had dropped their worth to a bear minimum. Buyers, under those circumstances, were always available, but I found it difficult, better say useless to part with them at such a loss. We still had Patrick's future to think about it and our own.

There was also my pride, or better to say my arrogance; it had conquered my life and blindfolded me to better solutions, such as to approach Mauricio for help. Likely with the factory's backing and the assets the partnership owned, it would have been possible to obtain a loan from the bank. Surely Mauricio would have said yes, but not first asking, "Why do you need so much money Myriam?" Not ready to share John Paul's illness not even with my husband, let alone with Mauricio, I kept quiet.

In that frame of mind I took what seemed a simple way out; get the cocaine to France and sell it to wealthy people in Cannes. Entrapped in my own web, I had not been able to see what was so clear presently. Too late I told the truth, yet no one from the French justice system seemed to believe me, or care and here we were now locked in a cell in a far away land and no one at hand to help us.

Helpless and contrite I reached out to the Lord. He had to be near. If I could only learn to walk with Him again, along the way, I could find His forgiveness; perhaps my husband's too and more importantly my son's. Momentarily I was appeased by this thoughts, save for I didn't hear jingling bells, or choirs of angels singing the Hallelujah for my homecoming.

No, but in my rapture I saw John, Patrick, and John Paul seated by my side in a very strange place and heard my husband distinctly say, "Don't worry dear; everything is going to be all right. I love you, and understand." Likely in an effort to pacify my intellect, my subconscious expressed what I wanted to hear.

My regret was sincere but it came too late. Even so, I recorded my thoughts for when I could connect with John. He had to know that the woman he married years ago, the one he totally trusted, still existed. Yet I knew John would never condone my fault, but perhaps there was a chance he would forgive me.

With this in mind, I re-entered my captivity situation, "No one will review your case until after the holidays." I remember one of the investigators stating this fact. Consequently I just had to wait until then to learn how things will work out. So when the next morning the investigators came back, my heart jumped with optimism; our case surely was evaluated and they were bringing the good news of my son's release!

What developed was not even close; "Detainees can't remain at the city's jail for more than 24 hours," the bully one said in fairly good English, an overnight improvement perhaps, and then added, "You will be now taken to the city's penitentiary where you will wait until a judge decides if your case will be tried here in Perpignan, or sent back to Nice." No further explanation, nothing, except that seconds later he rudely ordered us, "You need to pick up your belongings from the front desk, you are coming with us now."

John Paul didn't move, he had something else in his mind and annoyed spoke, "We haven't had anything to eat since the moment of our arrest. Is starvation part of the punishment or what?" Food of course, it was the least of my worries, but my son was a hungry young man and needed nourishment. Surprised I saw that J, P.'s request was accommodated. Black coffee and a couple of buns were brought and moments later we were escorted to their vehicle.

We had no idea of what was in store, but I had the feeling that we would be facing a possible separation, so before it happened, I wanted to say something, explain more. Yet it was John Paul who in Spanish spoke first. "Mom, we really don't know what is up ahead. Since you have gone this far just to help me, I now have the obligation to assist you. I thought about it last night. I'm going to retract my first testimony. In the next one I'll declare myself the guilty one."

My eyes were almost out of their sockets with the shock, and remained silent while I tried to collect my thoughts. "Oh my Lord, don't let my son do this; John Paul can't take the blame for me." I first quietly pleaded with God, and then responded to my son, "No! You will not do such thing." I said firmly and covered his mouth, so that he wouldn't interrupt me.

"John Paul I understand. I know you are only trying to help me. God will bless you for your love and good intentions, but it won't work. It will only complicate matters, because I'll immediately declare what you are trying to do. I have already confessed my crime; the police have all the details, while you have none. So please honey, don't act hastily. Don't make me feel any worse than I already do. Promise me that you won't do it." J.P. quietly listened, likely thinking things over and said, "Okay Mother, I'll listen to you, but remember, you can count on me for ever."

I supposed our secretive talk irritated the policemen, because the mean one, in his unkind manner said, *Ferme la bouche.* Fresh in my mind the books I read about the French Revolution, the atrocities perpetrated in the name of the so-called revolution flared up my imagination and the fact that we had not seen a lawyer fanned the flame. What if in France, because we were foreigners, attorneys wouldn't come forth to defend us?

Senseless thoughts, but in my frame of mind and the lack of a legal counselor, anything could be possible. Somehow we had to prevent being forgotten, so I told John Paul, "Honey the Canadian authorities should be notified of our detainment. A legal contact such as this would provide us with some safeguard, perhaps even a way to inform your father of our predicament."

It was not over appealing that my husband should learn of our situation through a frigid phone call from a consulate official, but I accepted it. As for the moment it seemed to be the only way to reach out to him and for help.

J.P. agreed and told the guards, "We would like to contact the Canadian Consulate. That office will notify our family of our detainment." But our request didn't amount to anything. In few words it was explained to us that under French laws, a judge was the only person who could authorize outside communication, even with the consulate.

The drive to the new facility seemed extremely short. A set of reinforced iron doors opened and the vehicle went in. Before it stopped, John Paul reassured me, "Soon everything will be all right Mom. It's important you remain courageous and remember that France is among the seven most developed countries in the world. And necessarily has to abide by standards of international law, more so in a situation such as ours. It's not like we are in Turkey and we can be thankful for this, Mom,"

He told me smiling, reminding me of the scenes in the Midnight Express movie. "I'm sure once a judge reviews the case, he'll realize you are not a criminal. He'll understand your motives and in no time you'll be released. You just wait and see, Mom."

The door opened and I was order to descend; I embraced my son and kissed him good-bye. His words were the last I remember. Like a zombie I marched to a cell. The prison was very old and my stay there was just a blur. How many hours or days went by, I am not sure. Somehow, I had disconnected myself from everything.

Until one day my cell opened and someone said, "Get ready, you are being transferred to Nice." Like a robot, I obeyed the order. The prison officials escorted me to the patio, where, next to a police van, eight uniformed policemen waited for me. Inside the vehicle, I saw my son, handcuffed.

What a way to be brought back to reality! I experienced the same pain as before, as if a dagger had penetrated my heart. Seeing my son under these conditions, treated as a criminal, would be my worst punishment. John Paul sat in one grated compartment, caged like a wild animal. I was placed in another similar partition, with four policemen who sat in front and other four in the rear of the van.

The prison gates opened. Once the vehicle started to move, the lights and sirens of two escort vehicles, one in front and the other behind the van, flashed and squealed. The display of security and police force that surrounded the transfer was overpowering. To guard who, a mother, whose only transgression was to bring seven hundred grams of cocaine into French territory and next to her, sat her innocent son, who had nothing to do with the plot.

Any attempt John Paul and I made to have a conversation was immediately stopped. One of the guards banged his billy stick on the grates, to scare us into silence. Any questions we had were totally ignored. My son and I were treated as dangerous criminals; the French gendarmes' attitudes said it all.

Soon the van arrived at a train station where we were ordered to disembark. A lot of travelers bustled around us. We carried our previously confiscated luggage; each escorted by four police officers, we marched! "Make way!" our escorts barked their orders. I could not help but blush as we sensed the contempt stare from the onlookers. I suppose the number of police escorts attracted curiosity and gave them reason to suspect the worst, a mobster's team? Their disdain made me resolve to never prejudge anyone without first finding out all of the facts.

At last we boarded a train, walked through jam-packed compartments. The scornful stares from the passengers, made me wish the earth would open and swallow us. They didn't know us from beans, but all the same it was just too humiliating. We went from one car after another, and finally found vacant seats at the rear of the very last car. The relief we experienced from being out of public scrutiny, was short-lived. The first stop, at a very impressive railway station that read Marseilles, we were ordered to descend.

The police escorts held their billy clubs as we passed through large crowds of people, ready to ensure us clear passage. I could not help it, but my thoughts flashed back to my hometown in Bolivia, where we were highly respected. Briefly, I wondered how did it all come to pass?

My reflection didn't last long; I had to keep up with the fast pace of the policemen. My luggage seemed to weigh a ton; in fact I was having a very difficult time. It dangled from one of my shoulders to the other; sometimes I even dragged it trying to keep up with them. It was a winter cold day, yet perspiration ran from my forehead down my cheeks from the effort of trotting and hanging on to my suitcase.

John Paul tried to help me, but it was impossible, handcuffed as he was; besides he was having just as much trouble dealing with his own suitcase. The lack of compassion shown by the guards to a defenseless woman enraged my son. John Paul's face turned red in anger, and with his fists clamped together, lifted his arms ready to strike one of them. I saw it in time, "I'm okay John Paul. I'm okay. Please honey calm down," I told him walking faster, my heart ready to explode but I had to prove to my son I could do it, as I was afraid for his safety.

Somehow we covered the distance separating us from the other platform and boarded the train heading for Nice. John Paul and I sat next to one another, but any attempt we made to have a conversation was rudely silenced. The gendarmes, insensitive to our physical needs, ate their lunch, chatting noisily as if we didn't even exist.

The hellish journey finally ended. We were back to where we had started, except that our status was different. The manner in which we were treated, increased my concern, especially for John Paul. I had the feeling we would not find much understanding among the French people. Who, from now on, would be in charge of our destiny?

Apparently the French judicial system was still based on Napoleonic laws, proved by the experience in Perpignan: "One was considered guilty until proven innocent." I now wondered if their prevailing system was much the same as what I had read in *Papillion*. Arriving at the terminal in Nice, the eight escorts were replaced by a new set of guards, who escorted us to a waiting van.

Once J.P and I were well secured and it started to move, the sirens and flashing lights screeched and flashed just as before, heading for our final destination: prison! No longer fearing any reprisals I decided to talk to my son, but again it was John Paul who took the initiative, "Mom, you don't have to worry about me. I'm going to be fine and I will keep my promise. God knows I'm innocent. So eventually I will be cleared."

He then smiling added, "It's you I'm worried about. As soon as possible we need to know what rights we have, and for starters, if we will be able to communicate with each other. Next, the Canadian Consulate has to know of our detention; it's important we establish this contact. Lastly we need to have the advice of a lawyer." The vehicle stopped and I was ordered to step out. I had no more than a second to respond to my son, so I nodded, but I managed to rush to his side and through the grill kissed his forehead.

Maison d' Arret du Nice, 1986

With my son's words still echoing in my ears, the tears I had repressed while we parted now ran freely down my cheeks, as I walked away from the van. My heart was broken, but this time I was not going to let my mind wander away from reality, much had to be done. Mechanically I followed the four policemen who ushered me into a building, while the van with my son drove away. Where? No one had bothered to inform me.

The file with my personal data was handed over to a clerk and I couldn't help but notice the different atmosphere here. People chatted and laughed among themselves, they seemed almost humane. As the clerk opened my file, he surprised me when with a smile he said, "*Buenos dias señora*," and still in Spanish continued checking my personal data. After the dreadful journey, it was a welcome change. For a moment I imagined being at the front desk of a *posada*, where a very diligent clerk waited on me.

The dream was short lived; someone else directed me to another office where I was put back in my place. I was photographed, fingerprinted and given a prisoner's ID, as "*Madame Del Castillo Myriam; Spouse: Arthur, John. No D'Ecrou* l69901 F1. *Maison d'Arrêt du Nice, Batiment de Femme.* Finished with the formalities, a large manila envelope was produced and all its contents emptied, shown to me, only for verification purpose. My wedding ring, two more rings, my watch and some other jewelry, also the American currency, all seized in Perpignan and retained now by the clerk for safekeeping.

He then in broken English told me, "The American dollars will be converted into francs and deposited into a prison's account in your name for future *canteen expenditures.*" Even exhausted as I was, the last words sounded out of place. In Spanish *cantina* happened to be an establishment where people ate and consumed alcoholic beverages.

I was flabbergasted, but I didn't have it in me, to ask, "Do you mean to tell me that people detained here, are allowed to buy drinks?" A strange way to run a prison, but we were in France. Perhaps for French people this was perfectly normal. I already had seen French officers drink on the job, so hey, why not if prisoners did too!

Somehow the confusion that dominated my brain evaporated and I ask, "Would it be possible to allocate part of that money for my son? His name is John Paul Arthur. He is also detained, brought to Nice with me, but I don't know where?" "Sure, there will be no problem. I'll take care of that," the agent answered making some notes.

The formalities seemed to have concluded, because the two females dressed in white uniforms that until then had waited aside approached and told me to follow them. Silently guarded by them we went into an older building. Walked through a shadowy passage, the overhead surface curved, a type of architecture I had seen in old churches and monasteries. Radical changes had taken place here since that now together with the barred gates that opened and locked behind us, gave me goosebumps.

We stopped in what seemed to be a storage room. One of the guards for the first time and with a heavy French accent addressed me, "Your suitcase will remain here, but you can choose a few items for you daily use." Still in some kind of denial, I didn't ask anything, I simply followed their instruction and chose what I thought might be necessary.

Next, I was ordered to undress and while I remained in the nude, all my clothes were examined just as before. This stripping business was just too much; not even in the privacy of our home did I exhibit myself in front of my husband. Thankfully the body cavity search was not performed this time either.

Over with that part of their agenda, I was handed a plastic basin, a glass and a glass bowl, and some cutlery, "You will be accountable for these items; they are for your personal use in the cell." Much lighter now, I continued in what seemed a never-ending walk. More gates were unlocked and locked right behind us; it would be a futility to try and leave the premises without those keys that hanged offensively from the guard's belts.

We entered a newer building, where another barred gate was unlocked and a flight of stairs came into my view. The journey's end seemed near and with every step I took, I quivered in fear. The staircase ended in a long hallway, on each side of the corridor I saw about fourteen identical doors. I was directed to the one in front of the landing, only a spy-hole broke the solid still red panel, ostensibly to peek inside, because one of the guards before she unlocked the double bolted lock, proceed to sneak a quick look.

Seconds later, the heavy iron door clanked shut behind me. The thud of the double bolts being locked hammered in my brain, tearing me apart. It not only deprived me from my freedom, but also brought me closer to a different reality. I was now locked in a prison cell as a criminal. Half paralyzed, I clung to the iron door, as if by a remote chance suddenly it would again open to let me free. Gradually, I let go of the door. Slower yet, I turned around and I was faced with three women in a very small cell.

The crowded and minute cubicle was distressing. No more than 14 feet wide x 16 feet long with a smooth cement floor. The two narrow beds sided to the left and right walls barely fitted, a sink mounted in a pedestal stood by the foot of the left bed and a small mirror above it. Beside this was the toilet bowl, somewhat hidden by a sheet that hung as an improvised curtain. A two by four-barred window, shoulder height facing the door, was the only source of fresh air. Underneath, separating the two beds stood a small table and two chairs. On the right hand, by the door, a bunch of clothes hung in a niche that simulated a closet.

The three women who had been sitting on the beds, got up, to greet me, or hit me? I was not sure. Frighten, I lost any perspective. The thought I could be imprisoned with dangerous and hardened criminals dominated my mind. Suddenly, I felt faint. Unable to get enough air into my lungs I broke into a cold sweat. I supposed the confinement, combined with my anguish caused me to suffer a mild form of claustrophobia; as a child, even later as a grown up, I had experienced something similar.

Prompted by curiosity my newly found roommates came closer. Terrified I recoiled, but soon their attitude and a couple of kind words one said calmed me down and gradually I recuperated my senses. Odd, I even felt protected from any further inhumane treatment. Stranger yet, soon I found myself intensely sobbing in that same cellmate's arms.

To find only these sympathetic women, instead of the mobsters I expected to encounter, eliminated the previous ideas I had. Besides at this point, I could have cared less if these females had dreadful crimes in their pasts; all that mattered was that they had shown me warmth and some kindheartedness.

Their English was not the best, their Spanish not any better. Yet in a joint effort we overcame the language barrier. The oldest, the one who spoke kindly during my panic attack, was perhaps sixty and with a seemly German accent said, "My name is Inge. I'm from Germany, but I have resided in France for the past twenty years." The smile in her weather down face brightened it up a bit and once again, solicitously offered me something to eat and a cup of tea.

In no state to eat anything, I accepted the tea. The petite brunette that I could now see better, closer to my age, in French spoke next. I liked her intonation, even if I didn't understand much. As she noticed my puzzled look, rapidly repeated it in English, "I'm Danielle; Parisian by birth, but at a very young age my family moved to Cannes. I have lived here ever since," she muttered smiling, proud of her English.

The one no older than thirty, whose features looked Spanish to me but were actually Arabic, spoke last. In mixed English and French she said, "I am Josee. We were expecting your arrival, but we didn't know to which cell you would be assigned." She interrupted her talk, seemingly with something else in her mind. Her search ended when triumphantly she presented me with a newspaper's page saying, "Read this."

Taken aback by her rough manner compared to the others, shaky again, I took the page in my hands. The paper was from Nice, of course in French and dated January 3rd, 1986, over two weeks ago, Part that I understood, but not the rest."I can't read French," I told her.

So Josee read the article, translating it slowly as best as she could to English, "A Bolivian and French drug connection has ended successfully, thanks to the effective intervention of the police patrol in Perpignan. Myriam Arthur and her son John Paul, from Cochabamba, Bolivia, involved in this illegal trade were apprehended yesterday while trying to cross to the Spanish border; a third party Judith Castang was previously arrested in Nice. Their trial, will take place at the Court of Grasse at a future date."

This was a bombshell I didn't expect! If a newspaper in France printed the article, involving even John Paul, a corresponded journalist could easily reprint the material in Bolivian newspapers. The gossip would be awful; everyone in my hometown would know about our mishap. I closed my eyes, with the childish idea that by doing so, the thought, the fact and the possibility, would go away.

Obviously this was how my roommates got to know I would be brought to Nice. Apparently Judith was already here, because Josee taking again control of the conversation strongly declared, "I've seen Judith. I'm sure, she is the one who gave you away. It's because of her you were arrested." I had no idea what caused her to arrive at this conclusion, perhaps because an inmate herself; she could foresee things beyond my understanding, or even have inside information?

If reading my mind Josee spoke, "Almost everything is known here and a certain standard of conduct exists among inmates, whereby anyone who divulges a persons wrongdoing, is ostracized. I suggest you be careful if you have the opportunity to talk to Judith." I was confused, but her presumption together with what I was told by the police in Perpignan led me again to question my friend's loyalty. I realized I would need to speak with Judith before I arrived to my own conclusion.

Inge and Danielle, on a less serious note cut in and filled me in on the cell's evening routine. My arrival was a little after seven p.m. and two hours had gone by since; evidently it was now time to prepare the cell for night. Speechless, I watched as the three moved things around; the table and chairs were put next to the sink. At first I didn't see the objective, but soon my instruction was completed. Two mattresses were pulled from under the beds, one placed on the space in between them, would be Danielle's sleeping place and the other set by the door and the niche-like closet, supposedly was for me.

With some experience under their hats, they knew exactly what to do with the bundle left on the floor when I was brought in. It hadn't drawn my attention then, but now I learned: it was my bedding. Josse covered the mattress with the sheets and the blanket, while Inge wrapped a pillow that appeared from somewhere, with a case and my resting place for the night was ready. Inge and Josee had the real beds; I learned later that seniority gave them that right.

During the hustle, not a sound or a movement came from me. I just watched in wonder. Inge concerned about my detachment handed me another cup of hot tea, together with a small white pill, saying, "Myriam, this will help you relax and sleep through the night, but don't ever mention to the guards. It is forbidden to have any type of barbiturates or drugs in the cell." I thanked Inge for her thoughtfulness, but I only accepted the tea.

Once the rearranging concluded, to venture behind the curtain and use the toilette, the mattresses on the floor necessarily were stomped. Our room resembled more a can of sardines, with the four of us jammed inside. Intense, but not scary, given that I now knew no harm would come to me from the women. But the guilt and worries didn't let my body find any rest. How could I sleep, when the world I knew was gone?

My son's ailment, his imprisonment, the hardships he might be experiencing thanks to my stupidity was overwhelming. What if John Paul and I were forgotten behind the prison walls? No one knew where were except the gendarmes who arrested us, and we didn't even have the help of a lawyer. What if the French justice system was more like Turkey's, what then? I lay awake searching for something to keep me afloat while the other women slept.

Voices and keys jangling in the hallway stirred me. The women, awake now, began to bustle around. As the routine of my first day at *la maison* unfolded, the three kept the same civilized manner, even with the bathroom use. The curtain in front of the toilet was utterly a joke; it didn't give any privacy. In a zombie-like state while in Perpignan, I didn't have a clue how I dealt with my body's needs or anything else during stay there.

More alert now, I carefully walked towards the small sink to wash-up, but as soon as my hands touched the water coming from the faucet, I withdrew them; the water was unbearably cold. Startled I looked around for help. Danielle seeing my surprise told me, "There is no running hot water in the cells Myriam, but we have a way to solve the problem here."

She presented a couple of plastic pails and continued explaining, "We first gathered the liquid element and then heat the water with electric gadgets; these two belong to Josee. We can purchase them from the canteen, and other items too." While still talking she show me how. As soon the water was warm, each one took turns for a quick wash.

Only now I realized the use for the two plastic basins handed to me at my arrival, it was to facilitate my personal hygiene. Washed and dressed, I saw the morning routine unfold; the two mattresses and the night gear went back into hiding and the cell was arranged for the day. I tried to help, but unfamiliar with the practice, my efforts were useless.

By seven o'clock the door opened and two female guards in white uniforms, the garb used at the *maison*, stood vigilant by the opening. A couple of young women distributing food from a wheeled cart, with big smiles on their faces said, *"Bonjour."* Josee, all spirited, handed over the two large glass bowls she retrieved from the shelving under the small table, and one of the girls in charge of the catering poured hot coffee and milk into the bowls, while the other handed her some French bread.

As the door shut, Josee, whom I started to realize was a going concern, smart as a whip and even able to read my thoughts said, "In case you are wondering about those two? I'll tell you. The blonde is Sylvie and the brunette is Corinne. They are prisoners like us." I quietly listened, while through the back of my eyes, I saw Inge and Danielle get some utensils for breakfast and except for the basket with the bread that lay on Inge's bed, the small table held the bowls, the mugs and the rest. Inge and Josee sat at the edge of their beds, while Danielle and I sat on the two chairs.

Once breakfast was over and still as an observer, I saw dishes being washed in one of the basins and in a matter of seconds put away. Josee taking again her self appointed guide's role explained, "The cell has to be meticulously clean and arranged. You were very lucky Myriam; it so happens that you were placed in a model cell, shown regularly to outside visitors such as politicians, human rights activists and religious groups. Mind you this is set only as an artifice so that prison's conditions are seen in good light by those people." I suppose she was right, even if anyone should be considered fortunate of being confined within four walls!

At nine o'clock, a guard opened the door and said, "I'm Madame Gonzales. I am here to fetch Myriam." Distinctly a Spanish surname, the Madame title was the way we were to address the guards. The minute we left the cell and marched down the stairs, curious about her last name, I asked, *"Habla Usted. spañol?"* She nodded and smiling in perfect Spanish announced, *"La asistente social quiere verla en su oficina,* I will take you there."

Somehow I sensed Madame Gonzales was going to be an ally. I followed her into a hallway similar to the one we left; the difference here was that the doors had glass sections, instead of the solid steel panels. I was directed to one that read *Assistante Sociale.* The young woman that waited inside in very good English, but with a slight French accent greeted me with a bright smile on her face, "I'm Patricia. I don't speak Spanish but we can certainly communicate in English."

She offered me a chair, where I sat down, and she waited to proceed. From the file in front, Patricia read my personal data to verify if everything was correct. She then explained, "I'm not here to judge or absolve, but to assist all the inmates. What can I do for you, Myriam?" I immediately took her offer and inquired, "Do you know where my son is? Can I talk to him?"

"He is in this prison as well, at the men's side. You'll be able to write to him as often as you want, and visit him once a week, but only after a special permission is granted by *le Juge d'instruction.* To obtain this authorization you need to write to him. The decision is entirely his," Patricia slowly informed me, making sure I understood everything.

"Will it be possible to make a telephone call? I need to call my husband in Canada. He is in Quesnel, British Columbia visiting his parents, I have to let him know what happened to us. A collect call if necessary. May I please?" I was almost in tears as I asked. "That's not possible," she sympathized with me. Yet encouraged by her tone and friendly smile even if her answer had been negative, I asked again, "May I call the Canadian Consulate, then?"

"No, I'm afraid not. No phone calls are allowed to inmates. However, if you want, I can contact the Canadian Consulate on your behalf." It seemed I had reached a dead end. The only way I could connect with the outside world was through her. Left with no other alternative I had to tell Patricia my problem and have her notify the Consulate, momentarily leaving my son's illness out from the account.

Patricia looked up in a telephone directory, found a number and placed the call to the Canadian Consulate in Marseilles, the regional office for Southern France. She spoke in French, thus my eagerness to learn the result of the dialogue had to wait until the end. Once *l' assistante sociale* hung up the receiver, she informed me, "Mr. Tony Andrew, the Vice Consul has promise to give notice of your whereabouts to your husband. He has also said he will come to see you and John Paul the minute his workload allows him."

I don't know what exactly I expected from this phone call, but since nothing concrete had come up, discouraged I told Patricia, "I'll likely need a lawyer. Will you help me find one?" I thought this time my request would lead me into the right path. So when Patricia handed me a couple of sheets of papers with a list of names, I didn't have a clue what to do with them. I just stared at the papers with a blank look on my face.

Moved by my perplexity, she added, "Myriam, personally I can't suggest any lawyer. It's against regulations. She then took the papers from my hands and in sequence handed them back to me. "All I can tell you is that in this page, you will find the names of Legal Aid lawyers, paid by the state. This other one has the list of attorneys, paid by the clients. Their price varies; it's normally arranged between lawyer and client," the young lady patiently explained.

She certainly had to be part of the prison system, but her kind manner to some extent erased my earlier distrust. So, inquisitively I continued with my questions, "Can I write to my family?" "There will be no problem with that," she said obligingly. "My address book is in my suitcase left in storage, may I have it back?"

The dilemma was soon solved as she promised, "I'll take care of it right away. You'll have it back this afternoon. Is there anything else you need?" Patricia said looking at her watch. As I shook my head, she added, The *directrice* (warden) has requested I read and explain the rules and procedures of this precinct. They needed to be followed to the dot if you don"t want to get in trouble. She unfolded some papers and began to read a long document.

"The female sector of the *maison d' arret* is only a small detention center where inmates wait for their trial. Normally only two inmates should be placed in each cell, yet presently there are four and five, making the confinement very difficult for prisoners as well as for guards.

"Any irregularity or inmate uprisings are severely punished, in isolation when necessary. If a detainee is found using, or in possession of drugs, an investigation is conducted and all visiting privileges suspended, followed by a full report sent to *le juge d'instruction*, which always has a negative bearing on the trial. Only female guards are in charge of the surveillance, they should be addressed as *Madame*. Male guards are called to the wing only in case of uprisings.

"Inmates who come from a country other than France are entitled to an elementary French class along with basic arithmetic. The program was established by the judicial system, to benefit prisoners who successfully finish the course; a three-month's remission in the sentencing time is granted. The same teacher offers classes in crafts in the afternoons

Items not provided by the prison such as personal toiletries, writing material, envelopes, stamps, fruit, cookies, milk, sugar, coffee, tea, butter, soft drinks, cigarettes and beer, (only two cans per inmate) can be purchased through the *canteen* once a week. The cost of the products is deducted from the prisoner's trust account. "You opened one as you came in, right?" I nodded, all this information was overbearing. Yet I had to laugh at myself about my interpretation of the *canteen* thing. Now I knew exactly what the word meant. It was a place where you did all your shopping, including the beer, so I was not too far fetched after all!

Patricia continued giving me some other details. "Inmates who do not work have showers twice a week. You will be later notified of the schedule. Outside shop owner sometimes provide piecework; it is an inexpensive way for merchants to obtain cheap labor, paid by them. Unfortunately, just a small number of inmates participate in this type of work because of the limited workshop space."

Patricia paused for seconds, wanting to know if this would interest me or not or not. I listened to her lecture attentively but the explanations didn't mean much to me. I was still confident that my detainment would only be temporary. Just the same, wanting to be in the prison's good side, I told Patricia, "I'm interested in both of the classes, as well as in the piecework."

"Very well then, I will sign you up for the school activities and your name will be kept on hand for future work." She handed me some papers, which I immediately signed. Patricia then concluded my audience.

When I was brought back to the cubicle my cellmates, curious about my interview with the social worker, bombarded me with questions. Especially Josee, who definitely seemed to want to be in control, "What did she tell you? Were you allowed to talk to your husband, or your consulate?" Of course they felt free to ask these questions, I had made them aware of all my uncertainties, myself.

"I'm allowed to correspond with my family." The last word just out of my mouth and Josee quickly informed me, "Myriam, it's important you know that all your letters will be first subject to censorship by personnel at *le juge d'instruction's* office. The mail is delayed for days, if not weeks. It's a way they use to spy on us." Since she seemed the one most versed in prison matters, continuing with her rhetoric she said, "About the permission to correspond with your son, there have been cases where this permission was not granted, but I do not see any reason for this to happen to you!" This time she had a positive inflexion in her voice. I hoped she was right.

As it appeared she was finished, I began to look at the papers Patricia handed to me, in search for a lawyer who spoke English or Spanish, but Josee, still very much involved with her role of adviser decided to speak up again. "Myriam, lawyers are very costly. One with those qualifications, probably will cost a lot. Do you have the money?"

Money! Oh yes, money. What I had in the prison's account was certainly not enough to pay for a lawyer, let alone a good one. I immediately thought of John, I knew that no matter how angry he was with the situation I created; my husband would do the impossible to send financial aid the moment he learned John Paul was ill and detained.

Sarcastically, I congratulated myself on such great thought, "Your husband is in Canada, you idiot. He doesn't have access to any immediate funds there. Besides, you don't even know when the news of your arrest will reach him. You require legal advice immediately; your son needs to be freed and start with the treatment right away, not in a million years." After this brutal rebuttal from my brain, my ultimate goal now was just find an attorney from the Legal Aid list and I told Josee, "No I don't have money; a legal aid lawyer will have to do." She laughed at my response. I believe she was under the impression I was loaded with the green stuff. I left it at that.

Still my expectations to find one with good credentials from this group were minimal. In my country all state appointed lawyers were inexperienced law school graduates, taking on cases as hands on practice, France had to be same. However I needed one, so I examined the list carefully and *Maitre* Elizabeth Grontier's personal data came to my attention. The entry, 'English spoken, ' next to her name was the key reason. I wrote to the judge immediately, notifying him of my choice, also requesting his permission to correspond and visit my son.

Writing to my husband was my next priority, but it had to be postponed for a while longer. Prison matters got in the way. It was 12 o'clock, lunchtime, and *la routine quotidien in la maison* had to be followed. The meal brought to the cell was in the same fashion as breakfast by Sylvie and Corinne; but it didn't even seem tempting. What's more, I had no appetite, but I joined my roommates at the table. The cell's size didn't leave me any choice, other than to stand in a corner. At the end of the meal, more experienced now I helped with the clean up. Everything was put back in place and the cell looked impeccable, as if only two inmates occupied it, instead of four.

Informed of a two o'clock outing to the courtyard called *promenade,* and it was only about one now which allegedly gave us enough time to relax beforehand. Easier said than done for me! My entire body was a compound mass of nerves and my mind was in a continual gallop. I had to write to my husband, yet because my brain was overloaded and ready to burst, I could not do it. I could not sit still. I needed immediate help, but I had no place to turn. So I paced the floor inside the minute cell instead and all I managed to do was cause some irritation with my roommates.

The morning promenade eluded me because of my interview with Patricia. I had no intention of missing the afternoon one; I was starting to feel claustrophobic in need of fresh air and some breathing space. A few minutes before two o'clock my cellmates began to get ready. One by one sought the privacy behind the improvised curtain. I was encouraged to do the same. "There is no bathroom facility at the promenade Myriam and the guards don't appreciate opening the gates, save in an emergency," Inge advised me, taking the role of a mother hen watching over her chicks.

Each got dressed in their winter apparel, while talking about the weather conditions outside. Josee looking with a smirk at my winter garments, impatiently said, "Myriam, the afternoon outings at this time of the year are extremely cold."

"We hardly get any sun there, the high walls surrounding the court prevents it. You will be very cold wearing only that," Danielle added in a lighter tone. I wore nylons, a warm but light cashmere sweater, wool pants and my leather boots. Also my well tailored winter coat, with fur on the collar and cuffs, which had already proven worthless in Perpignan, and a pair of leather dress gloves. From their looks I appreciated, it was a very smart wardrobe, but not the most appropriate in prison, let alone for a winter day. Unfortunately that was all I had. What did they expect me to do? Oh sometimes these ladies irritated me!

Promptly at two, a new set of guards unlocked the cells. All inmates who wanted to partake in the promenade were let out. It turned into a large crowd. As we descended the stairs I saw Judith; everything else disappeared from my view, except her. Josee's forewarning came rushing to my mind. "Soon, you will see your friend, but remember, she is the one that gave you away. Be cautious if you have a chance to talk to her."

Now I didn't know what to do. Would it be safe to approach her, or would it be better if I didn't even get near her? As soon as we were let out into the courtyard, fear held me back from immediately walking towards her, but my need to find out what took place that dreadful morning of December 31 was greater than any preventive measure. I had to talk to her! As I moved towards Judith, I noticed her paleness and the frightened look on her face. My heart pounded loudly; probably I looked just as scared as she did. In seconds I was walking by her side, asking, "What happened, Judith? Why did you give me away?"

She had tears in her eyes as she shyly responded, "Myriam, it wasn't that way at all. I didn't do any such thing. You have to believe me. I think the deal went sour because you were followed." Judith was convinced this was what happened, because of the way she was arrested. Apparently, the police told her that her house had been under surveillance, she assumed then that the police had been waiting for me.

Not one guard came to interrupt us; so we kept walking and talking the same as everyone else, while she related everything that happened from the moment we parted that fateful morning. "After we said good-bye at the car rental, I returned home and did some chores around the house." Judith's voice was shaky, but she continued talking. "Just before I left for the rendezvous, I went to the car and placed the cocaine under the back seat on the driver's side. I said good bye to Jean Pierre and my children and told them I was going shopping to the mall." The rendezvous was to take place there.

As Judith relentlessly explained the rest, tears began to roll down her checks, "At the mall parking lot, the two men that came to my house the night before, were waiting for me. When they saw I was alone, they inquired."

"Where is your friend?" "She had other matters to attend."

"Do you have the powder?" "Yes." "May we see it?"

"I got out of the vehicle and pointed toward the back seat, and as I was showing them the cocaine, out of nowhere two other men jumped in front of me, flashing police badges. The first two men fled, while I was arrested on the spot and taken to the police station for further questioning. There in a threatening manner I was told, "We are aware of the trafficking; your house was under surveillance. It won't be long before we arrest your husband and seize your home and car. We advise you to tell us the truth."

Intimidated by the officer's words and afraid for my husband, I couldn't help it Myriam. I had to tell them how I came to be involved in the trafficking and clarified that Jean Pierre had no knowledge of it. But I never told them where you were going. It wasn't I who sent them after you. You have got to believe me, Myriam. I'm sure you were followed."

It was not hard to understand her fright. After all, I had been afraid too. Neither one of us had any criminal background, Judith had feared for the safety of her husband and possessions. I could not really blame her for that. We were both in deep trouble now, and mainly because of me. She was maybe ten years younger than I, even if I had not forced her to participate in the trafficking; it was literally because of my influence that she became involved.

Since my confession to the police in Perpignan, I had not told anyone else about John Paul's ailment. Now I felt I had to clear the air with Judith. She had to know my tormenting secret, be aware that it was not just for money per say that I got her involved.

All out in the open now, she asked me, "Why didn't you tell me before?" "At the time I couldn't. John Paul and I weren't ready to share our tragedy with anyone. I haven't even told my husband. I planned to let him know as soon J.P. started with the treatment."

Silently I recapped her words and felt something didn't make any sense. I didn't believe the police were aware of my trafficking and would have followed me. Given away by someone I contacted myself? Not likely, I had considered the possibility before, but there was no logic to it. My sixth sense told me the problem originated in France. If it was not Judith who notified the police, it had to be someone she herself contacted who alerted them. In my view, the two men that showed up at her place the night of my arrival, had to be undercover policemen. Only one person could have set up the whole thing; it had to be Judith's contact!

Immediately I told Judith what I thought, that it was her friend who gave us away. But she didn't believe me. On the contrary Judith stood by her comrade's loyalty, stating that she was trustworthy and that I was mistaken.

Involved in our conversation, we didn't see it had not passed unnoticed; a number of women had their eyes on us. Unease with their curiosity, we decided to resume our talk another time and parted ways. I had failed to press attention to anything except Judith before, but now as I walked through groups of inmates searching for my cellmates, I examined my surroundings and from every angle I looked, everything was appalling.

What is more, the stonework on the walls at two sides of the courtyard, crowned with barbed wire, gave the place a lugubrious note. The approximately 8.000 square foot area was divided in three sections. Where Judith and I had walked, was the largest and farthest away from the building with hard-packed dirt, used by the residents' for their daily walks.

The portion connected to the building structure by a barred gate was under a tin roof and had cement floor. Four iron benches and a game table was the full décor of this sector, plus two clothes lines extended from side to side. In the smallest one, between the two partitions, some grass and a few plants made an effort to survive through the winter season.

The yard was not huge, but marching through groups of women, who coldly scrutinized me, gave me a chill. Best not to ever cross them, I told myself and walked at a faster pace to rejoin my roommates. Only to find a number of other inmates had gathered at their side. Mislead by my garments, they believed I was an outside visitor, a politician or a churchwoman.

When my companions told them differently, they wanted to get the particulars of my crime. Certainly not through me, I had no intention of telling them anything. However, Josee already had volunteered some information and now they tried to fish for more details. They could fish in another tank, because mine was empty; gossip was not my cup of tea.

At three o'clock, the first hour of the promenade ended. The guards rounded up the prisoners who wanted to go in and guarded them back into their cells. The outing continued for one more hour, I chose to remain. I needed to be alone and digest Judith's words. Confined in the cell with those three women for the rest of the day would not give me the chance, it would be exasperating no matter how kind and helpful they had been.

But the next hour proved to be beyond physical endurance, the bit of sun that until then shone at the courtyard, disappeared. Exposed to the humid wind blowing from the Mediterranean Sea, the temperature dropped to minus zero. At least that is how I felt, frozen to the bone, my winter clothes didn't help maters; I was shivering!

Every one who remained at the court seemed cold, but not as much as me. One of them even told me, "Your lips are blue." Probably so, for sure I knew that my fingers tips were white and ached. To keep my blood circulating, I marched around the court like a maniac, the same as the rest. By four o'clock literally frozen, I was glad to go back to my cell; the brutal chillness of the afternoon surely had damaged my brain!

Madame Gonzales who was one of the guards on duty, seeing how dreadfully cold I was, politely inquired, "Del Castillo, don't you have more appropriate clothing to wear?" It was odd to be addressed that way; something else I would learn to accept. When I shook my head, she promised to look into the problem and left.

Minutes later she returned and said, "Follow me." While she kept talking, we went downstairs to the end of the corridor, "The Warden has granted you permission to search for warmer clothes from a stack left behind by released inmates."

We entered a large room that looked like a workshop, where I saw the two young women who cater the meals. Corinne ironed what appeared to be sheets, while Sylvie slightly stooped, seemed to be having some difficulty with a sewing machine. In spite of this, she immediately got up when Madame Gonzales told her, "Sylvie, will you show Myriam the winter apparel available."

While choosing my new wardrobe, I noticed Sylvie said something to Madame Gonzales. Incomprehensible because she spoke in French, but her motions indicated she was frustrated with the sewing machine. Instinctively I said, "Perhaps I can help you?" Both looked at me in wonder. Then Madame Gonzales asked me, "Do you know anything about it. Do you sew?" "Yes, I do."

Relieved they let me intervene. In no time I had the problem solved; the thread had only been jammed. Sylvie, more solicitous now, directed me to a more varied stack of clothing, while talking to me in perfect English. When I returned to my cell, I had a few more warm pieces of winter apparel and a new friend.

At five o'clock the last meal of the day was served. I still had no desire for food. The state of my mind had a lot to do with it. Later when my companions seemed to have settled down, I had the stretch of the night to write to my husband. I couldn't put it off any longer; mail was picked-up at breakfast, Monday through Friday.

Likely the Canadian consul had already notified him, coldly saying "I just learned, your wife and son are imprisoned at the *maison d' arret du Nice*. I don't know much, but I'll try to find out more." No further explanation It couldn't be otherwise; the consul didn't know anything else. He had no inkling to the crime I committed, or my reasons. It was time I broke the news to John myself, but I didn't know how.

For a start, I pulled my mattress from under Inge's bed. It allowed me to have my own space and seated in a yoga position, I put into writing the thoughts I had ever since Perpignan. An eternity seemed to have passed, but actually it was only two days since our arrival to la *maison*, and eight, since our arrest.

I struggled trying to find the right words. How do you nicely tell the man you love, your husband that you have not only lied to him but that you also have deceived him in many other ways? How could I explain to this man, who for twenty-five years had given me his love and entire trust, that I kept from him something as important as his son's illness? It was not easy, but finally I found the courage to put into words the whole story.

My heart ached for John! My husband was going to receive the most dreadful news of his life by means of a simple letter. I knew that once he read it, my words would tear him apart. He would learn about our son's ailment and my dishonesty; the reasons why we were now both in a French prison. My deepest feelings went into the letter, but would my husband's heart be touched by the context, would he understand and forgive?

Following my written confession, I must have fallen sleep. I couldn't comprehend the next morning how this could be possible, after the hurt my letter would cause him. I suppose my body was just too worn out; it might have also helped that I released all that I had kept from my husband for far too long.

Another day went by, then two and three, and my awareness about life in confinement increased. The input from the three women in the cell was a strong guideline. I realized that some luck must have been left on my side after all, given that I was placed in this particular cubicle: clean and where the occupants were well mannered, unlike the others where everything was chaotic and the inmates were involved in constant quarrels.

The shortages were evident, particularly in what concerned our hygiene. Only working detainees had the privilege of showering every day, for the rest of the population the schedule was only twice a week. Mondays and Thursdays for even cell numbers, us. Guards chose which cell to open first. The call started at six o'clock in the morning, we had to be up by then or simply we would be skipped.

Our cell's turn came on my third day and the first door to be opened was ours. Forewarned beforehand, I was ready. Vaguely I remembered having a shower in Perpignan, where I was even given something potent to scrub my scalp to eliminate any lice I may carry. Imagine; how could I have forgotten!

I was not going to miss the chance to have a proper wash now, but I had just finished rinsing my hair when suddenly the water turned cold. Shivering and cold I got dress and went back to the cell. Where Josse half laughing, half apologetic lecture me, "You should never shower for more than ten minutes. A timing device has been set, which automatically kicks in at that time."

Prompted by the lack of running hot water in the cell and the limited time at the showers, my companions, who by now I learned were masters of ingenuity, found innovated techniques to resolve the deficit and the use of the electric doohickeys became multiple; either to have a quick wash in the morning and wash dishes after each meal.

Soon my roommates' lectures and coaching kept me at par with their knowledge, to where I was even benefiting from the refreshing spa-baths they had implemented in our cubicle. Squatted inside the large washbasin, use as a tub now, and aided by the small hand basin, I poured the pre-heated water from the pail onto my body; all performed behind the curtain for privacy.

Inmates also lack a laundry facility, so very democratically we carried out the chore in the cell. We appointed a specific day of the week to launder our garments; the small items were dry in the cell, heavier ones brought down and hung on the clothesline at the court yard.

My life at *la maison* was constrained but not perilous. I didn't experience any harm or threats. Nonetheless to share quarters with the three women from different cultures and walks of life was taxing. Yet it proved to me that the best in human beings surfaces when people are bound by tragic circumstances, at times the worst too.

Still my most fervent desire was to hide under a blanket and sleep until the nightmare was over. But this form of escape didn't come true no matter how hard I tried. Besides something else more powerful than my own misery worried me: John Paul's ailment and the damage that the deprivation he likely was experiencing would have on his health.

Just to continue living, even if I didn't want to, each day I forced myself to play make believe games. A good subject were the meals that in my game I pretended were prepared by prestigious male chefs at the *Batiment des Homes,* brought to our chambers by a well groomed chamber service.

The menus extravaganza started with breakfast, served at 7 am and brought countless choices; powdered milk diluted in hot water, and coffee that had gone through the ringer in a similar process, but thanks to my compelling imagination I turned it into an aromatic French cappuccino. On the side, came the sugar, butter and the well-known French bread. We could have an unlimited number; it had to do us for all three meals.

Lunch served at 12 o'clock, brought mind-boggling dishes, such as tripe, heart, liver, blood sausage, kidneys or squid; one specialty feature as the main course per day. Delicatessens I knew existed, but never before I had tried them. I believe because it was an exclusive trademark of *La Maison d'Arret du Nice.*

Occasionally more down to earth dishes were served, such as small portions of pork or beef cooked in tomato sauce and sautéed onions, a French stew, perhaps; all courses came with potatoes, couscous, carrots or peas and I was told that on special holidays, meals resembling more the repasts from the new world were served, such as small portions of beef stakes, or pork chops, even a small fish fillet, which I yet had to see!

The final touch came in the form of desserts. In winter, the season presently happening, dried fruit served in different styles tended to our sweet cravings; such as plums stewed in water with sugar, figs with no water or sugar, canned peaches in their juice and some other beautiful combinations. In warmer seasons I was told the treat was fresh fruit; considered a delicacy and sometimes we were even treated with ice cream.

By 5pm the highly trained cuisine staff probably had retired for the day, therefore supper had no major variations from lunch; heated leftovers were presented. At first all that my untrained taste buds could take was the French baguettes but hunger worked wonders, consequently bit-by-bit, as days went by in time, I learned to appreciate all.

My knowledge of the pen's routine also improved; I learned that the linen and towels changed bi-weekly were laundered at the men's subdivision. Our side's only specialty was the mending, performed by the two young women, Corinne and Sylvie, who catered the meals and also maintained the wing's common areas clean.

The piecework brought by external entrepreneurs didn't reach many; only ten or twelve inmates executed the work. The small *atelier* on the main floor restricted the space and the possibility to be part of the crew was remote if not impossible, as a result daily showers were out of my reach.

In an effort to break the cluster's daily gloominess, the outings to the courtyard were lifesavers for me. Monday through Friday, from 9 to 11 a.m. everyone was rounded up to descend. The morning excursions were mandatory; only inmates deemed to be sick, attending classes, or in working crews were exempted. On the other hand the afternoon outings set from 2 to 4p.m. were not compulsory and thanks to my improved winter gear, I benefited from the two daily excursions.

Surely some of my brain cells were one step away from annihilation with such a dull existence. Yet it's amazing what one's mind is able to endure while subdued by uncertainties, but the lack of communication with my son and with the rest of my family, in addition not having a lawyer, were specifics that bore down on me.

Nights were my worst, especially when everyone settled except me, but I survived the first night, the next, and the next. It helped to remind myself of the words my son said, "We have to appreciate that we are in a civilized country not elsewhere." Like in my country per example, where not too long ago I saw the dire conditions of the men imprisoned in Cochabamba. Compared to that penitentiary, this place could be considered a one star hotel!

On my seventh day at the *maison,* one of the guards that opened the cell in the morning said, "Del Castillo, you need to be ready by eight o'clock. You'll attend French and Arithmetic classes 'til noon. I'll come back for you, shortly." By now I knew I had been striped from my first and married names; I was now plain Del Castillo, as if enlisted in the army.

Even as dismayed as I was, I looked forward to attend those classes. Something else would entertain my mind, other than just my own thoughts! In addition I wanted to learn the language. I was becoming sick and tired of people having tête-à-têtes around me and not understanding a word they were saying. It would be to my benefit to learn French.

As she promised, at eight the guard came back to fetch me. I followed her downstairs, where the classroom was located. The minute I stepped in, I was attracted by the teacher's friendly smile, "*Bienvenue,* Myriam," she said in French and repeated it in English "Welcome to my class Myriam. My name is Claudette; I'm your French teacher."

She was probably in her late thirties and good looking. The dark blond curly hair and the few freckles on her face gave her a mischievous look. Compared to me, she was tall; I was only 5'2". I could see Claudette had a friendly disposition. It came throughout all her pores and even if she was the instructor, which meant 'from the other side of the fence,' I liked her. She received me into her class on equal grounds. I sensed it. She never looked down on me because I was a prisoner.

Among no more than twelve attendees, I saw Judith too. At first we avoided contact with each other, foolishly thinking that an intimacy between us could jeopardize a fair understanding from the law. Since no one seemed interested, some days later in between classes, Judith and I began to talk. It was then that I learned more about her situation.

"Yesterday I received a letter from my sister Martha and another from Steven; you remember him, he is my younger brother?" Judith said. "Of course I do." I responded while thinking about Judith and Steven. They were what people called, surprise babies. Judith's mom thought she was going through menopause when she got pregnant first with her and a year after with Steven. Later her parents separated and Elvira, Judith's mom, moved to the States with her three youngest children, where the oldest son and daughter were established. Economically they all did okay, but Steven was the one who succeeded in business.

Getting my attention again, Judith spoke quietly, "Martha wrote that she spoke with my husband after my arrest and that Jean Pierre was out of his mind, drinking heavily and having strangers look after my children. Concerned for his state of mind and anxious for my two kids, Martha and Steven have decided to come to see me."

"I'm glad Judith. Surely they will be able to put some sense back into Jean Pierre." Martha was Judith's oldest sister; all five siblings were very closely netted. Absorbed in my own grief, I had not given much thought to Judith's situation. Perhaps I still held her responsible for our detention at the French-Spanish border.

Aware now, I could not just ignore it. A strong voice hammered my brain aggravating my guilt telling me, "Do you realize what you have done? What have you accomplished? Nothing, on the contrary you have ripped your family apart, as well as Judith's.

Your son is in prison, because of you; there is no excuse for your blunder. How do you intend to solve all this chaos now?"

My anguish increased as time went by, two weeks and then three and still I had no news from my son. I so much feared for his health. I had not a word from my husband either; maybe he had decided to disown me. Or perhaps the message conveyed to the Consulate for John had not even been passed on to him yet. I wrote to my mother and sister but my letters were ignored. At least this is what I concluded from their silence, and most discouraging to me was that I still did not have a lawyer.

I confided in Claudette about my lack of news from John Paul. She had become my friend and understanding my concern suggested, "Mention your apprehension to Patricia, the social worker. She often goes to the men's detention center, where she has contact with other co-workers. It would be easy for her to find out about John Paul."

I followed her advice and talked to Patricia, who a couple of days later reported, "John Paul is doing fine, Myriam. He is well treated, the same as you. Besides he is a likeable young man, he won't have any problems." Neither Claudette nor Patricia knew of my son's ailment.

January 18th when mail was brought to the cell, I received a note from Maitre Elizabeth Grontier, the appointed lawyer I chose, announcing her visit for January 22^{nd,} at 10 o'clock. Following her announcement, I couldn't contain my edginess; after 22 days of detention at last I was going to see an attorney! The next four days my workouts at the courtyard were more like strenuous marathons, pacing and thinking.

At 10 o'clock that morning, a guard opened the door saying, "Del Castillo. *Votre avocat est ici.*" Escorted by her, I was directed to a small cubicle on the main floor, close to the first gate and next to other three similar partitions. Immediately I was ordered to remove all my clothes and while I stood in the nude, the guard searched through my garments. Why the hunt? I asked myself, as I had not gone anywhere and the visit was from a lawyer?

Once in the clear, I proceeded to a larger room where a young lady, probably in her early thirties and about my height waited for me. Her fair complexion was highlighted by an auburn mass of curly hair. A couple of crinkles in the skirt of her well tailored blue suit seemed to be giving her a hard time; she was stroking the area with her hand trying to smooth them out as I approached.

The Legal Aid lawyer lifted her head and her penetrating blue eyes inquisitively observed me until they made contact with mine. In perfect English, she then introduced herself. "Maitre Elizabeth Grontier at your service, Mrs. Arthur. Just call me Elizabeth if you please," she said smiling, extending her hand to shake mine. Everything about her impressed me favorably, even more the fact that she spoke English with none of the heavy-duty French accent.

Subsequently she asked me, "Will you please explain the reason why you need an attorney?" Collecting myself I went over of what took place the afternoon of December 31; calmly I told her everything, the plotting and the arrest. While she listened attentively, I saw her taking notes. When I got to the point of telling the reason for my crime, my son's illness and his non-involvement, I went to pieces and an unstoppable stream of tears poured down my cheeks, the topic was too painful. It tore me apart. "You see, John Paul is innocent and my concern is the effect this imprisonment, will have on my son's health."

Elizabeth, who until then only nodded, said, "Mrs. Arthur your offense is very serious. Under the laws in the Jurisdiction of the Court of Grasse, it will be treated with the utmost severity. Here, *les juges d'instruction,* in America known as District Attorneys, and the judges are dead set against the use of drugs. All traffickers are harshly sentenced, even more when it involves importation."

In more detail she explained, "Yearly, Nice is visited by millions of tourists from around the world, wealthy ones, as well as other less fortunate. The local government and officials have implemented extremely rigorous laws to protect the area from unscrupulous drug dealers!" Her words shocked me. I wasn't a ruthless drug dealer; they couldn't brand me as one, or could they? The lawyer's statement managed to frighten me more than what I already was. Up until then, I hadn't considered myself as a drug dealer, or that I could receive a harsh sentence.

Going over her notes, Elizabeth continued, "I believe your fault will be mitigated by the circumstances that pressured you into the actual crime. Your situation will have a positive bearing on your case." As she continued talking, the attorney even gave me reason to believe I was fortunate, "You are very lucky, Mrs. Arthur because the District Attorney assigned by the Court of Grasse to investigate your case is Mr. Benoit Clavier. He is one of the few sympathetic District Attorneys in this jurisdiction, who I happen to know well. He'll be the one to conduct the investigation; you'll be questioned by him."

Could I have some hope then? The fear I felt was less intense after her last statements. It was useless to worry about myself anyway. I now realized I had done something terribly wrong, even if my motive was to save my son; but it was over and done. In due time, I would have to face my punishment and accept it.

Settled with this, what I needed to find out now was what Elizabeth had in mind to do for John Paul's release. How could she speed it up? In case she hadn't seen the total scenario yet, I remarked, "I don't understand my son's imprisonment. In Perpignan, I explained to the police everything, the same as I've told you. I'm the one who plotted the affair, bought the drug and brought it in myself. I've never denied it. I'm the guilty party. Why, then, was my son arrested and still remains in prison?"

Her response was encouraging, "From your explanation, I find it very clear that your son wasn't involved in your trafficking. Therefore, I don't foresee any problems in having him released. However some formalities have to be looked into first. I'll start to work on them right away." Her affirmation was a relief! Finally the mistake would be corrected, and John Paul soon would regain his freedom! Silently, I thanked God and congratulated myself for choosing the right lawyer.

My son's innocence was an undeniable fact. Anyone in their right mind should have immediately seen it, yet something blocked the police investigators' sight. Perhaps the language, who knows? Yet it was very difficult for me to understand why his innocence had even been questioned, simply because he happened to be with me?

The lawyer's visit started a little after ten o'clock. Originally, she had intended to go and see J.P. too, but our meeting took longer than she anticipated. It was almost noon; visits weren't permitted at this time of the day. The guards' vigilance was focused in unlocking and locking doors for the meal distribution. Elizabeth, aware of the impediment, promised to call on my son, later on in the afternoon.

The attorney's assurance for my son's prompt release boosted my morale. I could even visualize John Paul back in Canada, reunited with his father and brother and John alerted of his son's ailment would move mountains, so that he would receive all the medical help he needed. These joyful thoughts helped lift some of my burden. The incarceration crisis I created for my son would soon be over.

Apart that Judith's incarceration needed to be also resolved. I couldn't hide from the fact that I was responsible for her situation too. From the attorney's words, I understood that the penalty for anyone charged with the importation of drugs, would be more severe. It was my duty to find a way to help her. In my first testimony in Perpignan, I didn't say anything incriminating against Judith. So I decided that at the inquest, I would add a word here and there to divert some of Judith's involvement in the offense, towards me instead.

Next time I was with Judith, I shared my thoughts with her, "Judith when I'm interrogated again, I'll say you knew nothing about bringing the drug into France. I'll also add that it was me who placed the cocaine with the Bolivian tapestries you ordered without your knowledge, and that I only disclosed the truth once you arrived in France, at which time I asked you to help me find a purchaser." The appreciative look on her face touched me more than her thankful words.

It was all ludicrous and certainly incorrect, but I had nothing else available to amend the wrong I encouraged her to do on my behalf. In no way was my intention to deceive justice for a gain. If there was any, it was only to relieve my conscience.

Still all the voids plus the lack of connection with my son and my family sent me into a deep depression. The abyss became deeper in the course of this phase; I felt as if I had been placed in a dark pit and the key cast away. Patricia's periodical reports on John Paul helped a little, but because the news didn't come directly from my son, I was not sure if her information was even truthful, or she was just saying anything that would appease me?

Even my mind started to play tricks on me and I thought the attorney's visit had only been a dream. Every night I woke up covered in cold perspiration, from terrifying episodes and always the same nightmare. I see my loved ones battling a storm; a ship-wreck is in sight and no matter how much I want to reach out to help, it is impossible, because I am in the process of drowning myself. Too many powerful realities fed my distress.

Monday through Friday unfailingly for the past twenty-eight days now, I'd stood by the door at the distribution of the last meal of the day, hoping for a letter from my son to arrive. Or at least a word from the guards, notifying me that my request to corre-spond with John Paul was approved, but I got nothing!

Despaired and frustrated and nowhere to turn for answers, I wanted to die; the easiest escape for me. Until this particular evening as the mail was handed out, one of the guards called my name, "Del Castillo, you have some letters here. It must be from your son, or do you expect interior mail from someone else?" she said laughing and indifferently handed me the letters. Of course I didn't have anyone else and the guard knew it, but she was one of the callous ones.

I'm sure my heart jumped out of my chest as I received the letters. There were three and certainly all from J. P. Delighted

I held the letters close to my heart, as if by this contact I was hugging John Paul.

Nothing was more effective at getting me out of my depression than the warmth I now felt by the simple touch of my son's letters which were a solace to my broken heart! I had hungered for news sent directly by him, so I now devoured his words. I even read between the lines to quench my thirst!

Letters from my Son

January 6, 1986

Dear Mom,

After we were separated, all I could do was pray. I knew how frightened you felt and even then, you were still more concerned about me than for yourself. I feel the other way around Mom. I'm worried about you.

How is your habitat? Are you alone in a cell, or do you share it with other inmates; the same as I do? Are you all right? About me, Mom, please don't worry. I'm a man and I assure you, I can look after myself. Besides, I have decided to take this episode in my life simply as a new experience. So, to make my temporary residence in this place acceptable, I'll pretend I'm here by my own choice. Let's say I've now entered a Monastery for meditation time. Ha, ha.

Unfortunately I don't have absolute solitude; three unexpected roommates share my cell Though they are kind and friendly, they don't appear to have very reputable references, but I'm sure with God's help, I'll learn to accept their company.

Frankie is a young person, maybe 20. I believe the motive for his boarding here is detoxification; some shoplifting to provide the means for his addiction was the reason. Jack apparently swindled a few people and got caught in the process. Yves, the last one has an outgoing personality. If you saw him, you wouldn't think him capable of being an accessory to an accidental manslaughter. He speaks Spanish and French and is willing to teach me French. He owns a game of chess and we've played a match or two already.

At the promenade, I call it playground time, I have met other residents. A few speak English, others Spanish. One of them is serving a 10-year sentence for murder. Quite a bunch, but don't worry Mom, I'm okay. Some have shared their stories with me and as I listened to them, I can't stop comparing your mistake and theirs. The good Lord knows you didn't do it out of malice. I'm sure He understands; if you did something wrong it was only because you were trying to help me.

Everyone I've met here has shown me nothing but sympathy. I wouldn't have thought that such a word existed in a place like this. They've even given me their good wishes for the weeks to come. I've the strong belief that everything will end well. God will see to that.

I hope the money seized from you in Perpignan was registered here. I've been told that even here it's of great necessity. Supposedly, to buy personal hygiene stuff, plus other things, I'm not too sure yet, what. I'll let you know the minute I find out.

I'll end now, Mom, I'm a bit tired; keep me posted. I love you, J.P.

January 8, 1986

Dear Mom, I'm desolate. I don't like to be without news from you. The very first day I learned I needed a special authorization to correspond with you and for the visiting rights, I wrote to Le juge d' Intruction to obtain it. Apparently every one who has family confined at the Maison has to do so, but no response, yet. I just hope it won't be long now. I worry so much about you.

Yesterday I had a great surprise. I'm sure you got it, too, Mom. In the morning I went to see Marvell, the social worker assigned to me. At my request she called the Canadian Consulate. From the contact I learned father was already aware of our mishap. How I don't exactly know, but from the consul's explanation to Marvel, it seems that one of Judith's siblings got hold of him.

In any event, it was Dad who contacted the Consulate, to make them aware of our situation. However, because he wasn't informed where we were imprisoned, father requested their help to find our whereabouts. The Consul stated his intention to come and visit us in a very near future, in the mean time one of their representatives from Marseilles will come to check on us. Dad obviously is going to be in permanent contact with them, until he finds out more. Isn't this great news, Mom?

I have been snooping around here and from what people have told me, it seems we won't know how long it will be before the authorities will even look at our file. According to them, it could take quite a while, unless a lawyer expedites matters. We requested one from the moment of our arrest; perhaps we might have a better chance now.

The same guys spoke highly of a Maitre Gerard Thibault. Apparently is an excellent lawyer, well known for good results, but unfortunately also for his high cost. I'm just passing this on to you Mom; after all, it is you who has to decide whom you would like to have for a lawyer.

Maybe the Consulate's delegate can give you some other names.

It is important that you know, that once we receive the authorization to correspond, we can write to each other in the language of our prefer-ence, the same goes when we write to the District Attorney, (who here is called Juge d' Intruction) and to the lawyer when we have one.

Something else I want to share with you Mom, I'm trying to get a job. Acquainted with one of the guys who cater the meals to the cells, I asked him, to put in a good word for me in the kitchen, but my roommates warned me, it will be difficult to obtain such a job, because our case involved drugs. I'm still going to try. I want to work. At least I'll be able to provide for my own needs, while I'm here.

Since I am now in a Monastery, I have to tell you the great things I have accomplished with the guys here. At first they were often bad mouthing God, some didn't even believe He existed, but now, after my preaching, ha, ha, I have changed their minds. One of them, Ives is even reading the Bible. Isn't this amazing? I'm starting to think that what happened to us has a bigger reason than just what we see in front of our eyes. Maybe we are here to touch people's lives. I believe with all my heart, that everyone in this place needs more understanding than punishment.

Though I must admit, I do have my ups and downs too, but, having my family's love plus God's, I'm able to cope with almost anything, it enables me to come out of my downs very quickly. Physically and otherwise, I'm fine. Swollen glands haven't bothered me. They are almost back to a normal size. All my love and God bless you. John Paul

January 27

Querida Mamita,

Every day without news from you drives me insane. I found the neglect and lack of compassion shown by the District Attorney to be beyond belief; and unfortunately he is the one who is supposed to investigate us? I wonder if he likes to torture people to make them confess where there is nothing to confess.

Seriously, I was on the verge of giving up hope, when only a few minutes ago, the social worker made my day. She told me, "John Paul, you have the permission." Mom, now we can write to each other whenever we want. Better yet, in a couple of days (this coming Thursday), we'll see each other again; apparently that is the day assigned for interior visits!

So, for as long as we are here, which I know, won't be for too long, I'll have the privilege to have a half an hour outing with my mother. Exciting, isn't it? I can't wait. You might have some new reports to give me from Dad and Patrick. I'm so anxious that I don't know what to do until then.

The first two letters I wrote to you came back for lack of the stupid permission. Did this happen to yours, too? I'm re-sending mine; I'm too lazy to re-write old news again.

My health, I believe, is holding on pretty good. My glands haven't bothered me, but last week, I had a sore throat and some fever. I feel much better now. I hope you don't have any health problems and you are looking after yourself, eating properly, and buying the necessary supplements from the canteen, right Mother? I know you too well, Mom. I know you'll try to save any money and go without many things, with the idea that I need it more than you do. I'll be very hurt, if I find out that you are neglecting yourself.

I love you, Mom. Can you imagine the joy we will have in a couple of days? Who knows, maybe, I will be even able to give you a hug. You should see me. I'm dancing with the excitement. My

*roommates are looking at me with their mouths
open as if I have gone crazy*

Bye for now. Love John Paul

I read and re-read my son's letters. The twenty-eight days of being completely incommunicado was no joke, a torture yes. My son's letters were most reassuring; he was fine. As well as one could expect in a situation such as ours and considering he carried the threat of the deadly illness. Yet, with no eyes on his tragedy, J.P. comforted me instead.

His cheerfulness was catchy. Even if I knew that he was only trying to cheer me up. Actually my son's imagination was exceedingly greater than mine; I was thankful he had such a gift and used it in a positive way. Treating the incarceration as a growing experience, it was just like him. John Paul's attitude would never stop surprising me.

Some of my son words from his last missive, intrigued me, "Father was already aware of our mishap. He is the one who contacted the Canadian Consulate, asking them to search for us." I could not help but wonder why the vice-Consul had not mentioned this essential part to my social worker. Was she, or he not well informed, or was it lack of communication from both parts? With no other source of connection with my family, it was vital that whatever message I received from my husband through the consulate be accurate.

Presently all was just guesswork but thanks to my son's letter, I knew some events were about to happen. For one John already aware of our situation will be demanding an explanation; an intimidating thought, but fortunately the belated letter would be in my husband's hands by now. The other events were more promising; the announced visit with my son for this coming Thursday, plus a steady flow of letters and visits with him.

I just could not keep the great news all to myself, so I made my cellmates aware. Josee and Inge, who visited their husbands every week, gave me an idea of what to expect and the setting. The visits run from 9 to 9.30 a.m. A short half an hour, hardly enough time to exchange a few words, but better than no time at all. I would not be the one complaining about it; actually I was thankful and excited. More so since Thursday happened to be in two more days!

The night before, like a child before a birthday party, I carefully looked through my limited wardrobe in search of appropriate clothes for the occasion. Every one of my roommates got involved. Josee, understanding my zeal, went as far as generously lending me a beautiful red silk scarf that suited perfectly well with the rest of my attire. I had chosen my light brown cashmere cardigan, a slightly darker pair of pants and a white blouse.

The selection was approved. I now needed to do something with my hair. I had it at chin length, slightly curled at a beauty salon when I was out in the free world. Here I made use of my ingenuity. In secrecy, I had asked Sylvie for an old pillowcase, explaining I needed to tear it into narrow strips to set up my hair in curls. Playfully she let me have one saying, "Make sure it goes unnoticed by the guards, they might think you want to hang yourself."

Later in the evening, I tore the fabric in about twenty pieces and then tied the strips in knots holding bundles of my hair, to set them up in curls. I got the idea from a movie where old grannies use it to curl their long hair. I did the same. Frivolity? Absolutely not; John Paul didn't need to see the real state of my mind, so in an outward show I spruced myself up to look my very best on my first visit to my son.

I finished the job around nine, time when the cell like Cinderella turned into our sleeping quarters. Mattresses came out of hiding; everyone got in their pajamas and got into bed. Josee's radio played music in the background for a short time, while we each spent a couple more hours doing our own thing before the lights went out.

Normally I studied. Claudette, who had seen my interest in learning French, lent me some school material, but this night I left the books aside. I had something more important to do, answer my son's letters. So many things to say, questions to ask, the allotted thirty minutes for our visit, was not enough to even begin to scratch the surface.

Carefully, I re-read my son's letters, and putting some sort of order to my madness, I covered most of the important points. Later we could use them as a reference. My roommates were ever so quiet. They must have sensed I had a full platter and they contributed with their silence. I was very grateful.

January 28,

Dear Son,

You will never image the relief I got after I received and read your letters. Yet, I have to ask you to please forgive me; I was either brainwashed or brain dead because when the social assistant, told me "No letters to your son, until the Judge gives the authorization," I accepted it and didn't write to you. To deepen the problem, I was not even notified our communication was instated.

My hope was drained too. I thought the District Attorney had decided to throw the key away and forget about us, until today when your letters arrived and proved my assumptions wrong.

Now I'll try to be short and concise in all I want to tell you.

1. - We needed a lawyer quickly, but with no money to engage an attorney privately, I looked for a public defender. The one I found Maitre Elizabeth Grontier, nominated by the Judge per my request has recently been here. My reason for choosing her was because she is fluent in English. I have confirmed it personally, after she came to see me and I talked to her.

Furthermore, my choice turned out better than what I expected. Once I explained all the facts of my offense and that you had no part in my wrong doing, Elizabeth understood your innocence! Our attorney will right away start working on your release; you probably are aware of all this by now. January 25ve was when she came, and had in mind to visit you the same day, only in the afternoon, did you see her?

2. - About your father, I wrote to him. It was the most difficult letter I have ever written, but somehow I got the courage and told him everything. Please forgive me for this too, sweetheart, because I even told your Dad the secret we were keeping from him. I didn't think it was wise to keep it between us any longer; it was imperative he knew. He will be able to do more for you, aware of the truth.

3. - I'm fine. You don't have to worry about me in that aspect. I've actually been placed in the best cell, it's the show room at the Maison. It came along with three good roommates; they have been very kind to me.

The imposed incommunicado treatment we went through was the worst part. My worries surmounted, of course; you being my main concern. I even asked Patricia, the social worker here, to check your situation with her colleagues on your side. Supportively, she gave me periodic reports. I can't complain. Truthfully people here have been good to me as well.

Now John Paul, I need you to promise me something very important for my peace of mind. You need to always be truthful when it comes to informing me of your health, no matter what. Please don't ever hide anything from me, thinking that what I don't know won't hurt. It doesn't work that way! But if I have your word, only then, I can assure, you I'll keep calm. Okay!

Likely you are already aware of the French classes available for foreign detainees, if you aren't, see that someone gives you the information on this. Right now, your mother is one eager student. My goal is to learn the language, so that I can understand what people are saying around me, instead of thinking they are talking about *me. My teacher's name is Claudette. She is an awesome person and I have her friendship now.*

You will receive this note after our visit and probably I'm repeating myself, but bear with me, son, I'm just too excited and only trying to make sure I don't forget anything. The half an hour we'll have for our visit won't be enough to cover much.

Love you, Mom.

My nightmares and worries were not mentioned; John Paul had enough on his plate, no need for him to have more concerns.

In my stress-free life, I'd never given a thought before to people who could be unjustly incarcerated. It had no impact on my life, but I had the pre-conceived idea that whoever ended up in prison had to be a criminal of sorts and deserved the confinement. Now, my son and I were locked up! Except that John Paul was innocent and I was not a criminal of sorts. At least I didn't think I was. I had committed an offense true, but this should not typify me as a criminal, or would it? All was just too disconcerting and with so many things on my mind, I ended having another restless night.

In the morning, my heart pounding loudly, I stood behind the door ready to go and visit my son. Next to me Josee and Inge, who also were going to see their husbands. At nine o'clock, the door opened, but only the two were called out. If some one would have hit me with a bat, it might have hurt less. Robbed from my desire to see my son, again, I felt choked while automatically tears ran down my cheeks.

Ever since our arrest, whenever I was frustrated my only escape from the cruelty of my situation was through a cascade of tears. In between my sobbing, I managed to ask the guard, "Why am I excluded? I understand I have the authorization from the judge to visit my son. He will be expecting me." "*Votre nom, il ne pas dans c'est liste.*" That was it. With no further explanations she shut the door and left.

Everything in prison was hard enough; the language barrier, made my situation even more difficult. I felt in limbo and to be denied the right to visit my son, when supposedly the permission was granted, was hard to understand. It made me wonder if I had any rights at all.

I still found it difficult to accept that as an outlaw I had no rights. I had lost them the moment I infringed the law, no matter my circumstances. The rest of the day, I spent in complete despondency. It would not be until a couple of days later that I learned what happened. John Paul's next letter provided me with the details.

January 29, 1986

Dear Mom,

I can't understand this system. It sucks. How could they do this to us? Yesterday I didn't write to you as I normally do because we were supposed to have seen each other. I was saving everything to tell you in person. I believe we were excluded, thanks to the negligence of someone at the Wardens' office.

The guards tried to tell me, it was because the big heads, the one in your wing and in mine didn't know the permission had been granted, thus didn't give their okay. Of course a childish excuse, it was the social worker that originally gave me the information. So, if she had it, how could it be possible that the big honchos of the prison not know anything?

Of course they knew, the problem probably came from the neglect of some insignificant clerk, who didn't bother to add our names to the list. You know me too well right, Mom? At first I was so angry and my anger made me hate these people. More calm later, I was able to pray for them instead and much later even able to forgive them for their stupidity.

I know enough now that I'm going to make sure that next Thursday under no circumstances we'll be omitted and left out again. I'll be on their case. Reminding them every minute, in writing and verbally, I suggest you do the same, OK.

Now, I have to tell you something else new. Changes are happening around here left and right. For one, I was moved to another wing, which I found puts me closer to you; shortly I'll tell you, how I know this! My new cell, even if it's smaller has more privacy; the toilet is divided from the rest of the cell, by a half wall. We are now only three in the cell, instead of four and there are two night tables, how do you like that?

I'll get along just fine with my new roommates. They seem to be more on the intellectual side. One of them is an older gentleman from Yugoslavia; the other one is a young chap from Nigeria. This change happened because I'm studying French, and the teacher wants all the students grouped in one specific area.

Here comes the best part, the communal shower area for this wing is strategically located. The last time I was there, by pulling myself up to the windowsill, I was able to see your building. Someone enlighten me on this aspect; you are at only twenty five, maybe twenty meters away. Mom, we are that close. One of these days I might be even able to see you. I'll keep you posted.

It's bedtime now, time to say good night Mom, may God be with you always; love you. J.P.

Jan 30, 1986

Dear Mother,

First, my cold is now completely gone, and no swollen glands so please stop worrying. Second, I'm happy to hear you've found a good lawyer, Maitre Grontier, even if she is only a state-appointed lawyer. I'm looking forward to meet with her. Yes Mom, I received your letter, at least that part of the authorization is working, but no, she has not come to see me.

My French is coming along splendidly; the program is helping me a lot. I'm one of the most dedicated students, the same as you. The class is full of people from different parts of the world; I'm even learning Chinese. I'm sure you are doing just as well. I don't like to hear you say, that you are too old to learn. I know you are smart and still young. So, no excuses, Mother. Apply yourself and you'll be speaking French, as a native of this land.

Mom I want to say something that I notice and it's been bothering me. You don't have to be ashamed of anything you've done. The circumstances, for which you are in this place, will never change the fact of who you truly are. The Lord knows it, and don't you ever forget it.

Something else I've perceived while reading your letter, it's that you sound depressed. Please let me know what it was that brought this negative mood in you? We are fighters; "We don't drown in a glass of water," remember Grandpa often said this phrase? So please Mom, don't dwell on that emotion. If it's a legal matter that troubles you, better let the lawyer know.

Or if it's something an inmate said to you, be aware that not all the people around us are as

228 | MYRIAM ARTHUR

good, or as truthful as we are. I've been told that there are some, who to have a better rapport with judges or wardens, can even invent lies regarding inmates' cases, I hope nothing of this sort has happened, but try to keep this always in mind.

I'll write to you again tomorrow.

Love you, J.P.

January 31

Dear Mom,

Are you feeling better today? If I may, I have a suggestion to make. Please, stop worrying so much about me. I'm fine, though to some extent disappointed, because the lawyer hasn't come to see me yet. I supposed she will come sooner or later, I prefer sooner, but will see.

I have something specific to ask you today; you need to have the strength to continue forward. We must remember constantly that even if there are people with fewer challenges than ours, there are also others who have immeasurably more tribulations. Some, who have lost loved ones, their possessions, but by the grace of God they've learned to start a new life. Job is one great example of what I'm talking about. We must forever have him in our mind.

You've always have been a good mother for me and Patrick, also kind to every one who came to you in need of help or advice. Don't forget this Mom and keep a smile on your face while we go through this trial. It won't last long, I know.

For a change, I do have some good news to give you. Some of the inmates, with whom I shared a bit about our case, told me that we shouldn't worry too much about it. According to them, it's straightforward and bears no complications. Their thought in the matter is that in no time I'll be out of here. Now about you, taking into account your background they believe, Mom, that justice will not be too harsh on you.

They seemed to know what they are talking about. They have been in and out of the French Judicial System and know what to expect on a trial. I'm sure God will see to that too. So don't believe one hundred percent what the lawyer told you. By the way, she still hasn't come to see me.

I've been keeping myself quite busy here, working on family portraits for some inmates. I've become very good with my work and I'm, not bragging about it Mom. I even get treats in exchange, like chocolates and pop; especially from one, his name is Charlie. I intend to work on one of you now, if I can't see you in person every day, I will see you in a copy of you.

Guess what I been thinking of a lot lately? Of course you don't, so I'll tell you. It would be good, if we all moved permanently to Canada. In two more years, Patrick will start college and what better place than Canada? Of course, this is only an idea floating in my mind. It'll have to become the common desire of the entire family, not only mine to put it in to place. Let me know your opinion on this, okay?

I must say bye for now. With all my love, I wish you a good day and a very peaceful night. Love you, J.P.

February 1,

Adorada Mamita,

It's Monday, and I didn't receive your weekend letters. My days are completely spoiled when this happens. It's hard enough as it is, but to be deprived of the only source of satisfaction we have around here, doubles the boredom.

It certainly wasn't because you didn't write to me; I know this wouldn't happen. We've promised to write to each other every day, even if it's only a few lines, I'm keeping the promise, as I am sure you are too. I tried to remain calm, but it angers me to realize that we are in the hands of incompetent people, who could care less about the unnecessary stress they caused us. I better write about something else, before I become more frustrated.

How about if the subject is the showering situation on your side, I'm curious. Here, we are scheduled to shower only twice a week, unless one is a part of a working crew. I'm still hoping to belong to one, even if it's only for the extra showers. No such luck yet. You know how much I perspire, so I stink if I don't shower everyday.

By the way, today was my day to get sparkly clean and guess what? I again had the chance to peek through the window and I confirmed my original finding. You are at less than twenty meters away from my peeking throttlehold and I clearly made out the window on the second floor, the one next to your cell and sided to the stairs.

You are probably asking yourself, how do I know all this? I'll tell you, it's very simple. An inmate, who works in maintenance and does some repairs on your building, explained the layout of your floor plan. I have the feeling that it would not be difficult to see each other; perhaps even be able to exchange a few words from window to window. Mondays and Thursdays are my showering days; normally around 8 a.m. We must try and have a bit of fun.

Make sure your name is on the list for this coming Thursday. Just remind the guards ahead; we don't need any more stupid surprises again. I don't have much more to tell you Mom, except that that even on my moody days just to think about Dad, Patrick and you, helps me get back in shape.

Love you Mom. J. P.

From the day my son and I started to correspond, we wrote to each other every single day. Sometimes long letters, others short but normally never missed a day while we remained incarcerated. We both tried hard to lift up each other's spirits. I'm sure John Paul sensing how deeply embedded I was with my guilt, tried his mightiest to entertain my thoughts with positive words and with his artistic creativity.

The cheerful characters that he drew and sent in his letters brought me not only encouragement, but also optimism and even laughter. Other times he sent some of his more serious drawings; all of them beautifully inspired.

Assured by my son's letters and by own inquires, Thursday February 2nd, I knew my name would be on the list, and the night before the same as the previous week, I prepared myself for the great occasion. After thirty-three days, finally I would be with John Paul. It didn't matter that the time was too short, or that our visits were only once a week; at this point what mattered the most was that I would be able to confirm with my own eyes the state of my son's health, even if it was only for 30 minutes. It's amazing with how little one conforms trapped in a situation such as ours!

A surveillant opened the door and after she established I was on the visiting list, well dressed and excited, I followed Inge and Josse to the small booths where the habitual stripping took place, nine other inmates participated in the celebrated search of garments. Once cleared, one guard took the lead in the parade, opening gates and steering us through, while the other, who marched in the back, made sure to lock them back again. As the procession advanced, I recognized the first part of the passage; it was in the newer area, which I had passed through when I arrived.

The walk then continued over to a darker corridor, into a much older building with discolored grayish color thick walls. While the floor, likely still had the original inlaid bricks that thanks to the ware and tear of time were now uneven; characteristics I saw in old monasteries or convents back home; which made think that this place must have been one some time ago and changed into a prison later.

It was all that my imagination needed to get into gear and rambled through time; to the dramatic stories these walls would tell, if they could only talk. When church and politics walked side by side, but conspired against each other to gain control of the power. How many lives must have been broken behind these thick walls, because of family feuds, or who knows what else? I shivered with the thought. It must have been awfully hard in those days.

Until I heard a voice, "Here you go again Myriam, thinking about the problems people had in the past; what about your own situation and your son's. Shouldn't you be thinking about what lays ahead for you, instead?" I reprimanded myself.

A few more paces and our group entered a more-illuminated area and I made out the visiting stalls, small and just as ugly as the rest. It didn't matter. In a minute I would be hugging my son. Wrong! The security glass placed between the male's side and the women's served as an impenetrable barrier and prevented any physical contact among the parties involved.

Disheartened, I resigned myself not to hug my son, but at least I was able to see him and through the orifices drilled in the glass hear his voice. Soon the background didn't matter anymore. I ignored the gloominess of the site; the deep scrapes on the walls, perhaps engraved by someone in more distress than us, still tacit reminders of where we were.

We both tried not to show our real emotions, the distress we felt; John Paul masqueraded better than I. Besides the sole fact that we were in front of each other gave us enough reason to be glad. At least while the moment lasted and simply enjoyed every minute of our visit. We talked and laughed, made plans for after our release from prison. I even tried to challenge some of my son's viewpoints, "John Paul, I understand your desire to remain in Nice, while my trial takes place, but I disagree with you," I strongly told my son, after he mentioned his idea.

"Mom, from the beginning I told you that things happened the way they did, because God wants me to be by your side and that is exactly what I'll do. I'll stay in France until you are out of here. I know it won't be long." My son's words came out from his mouth with such zeal that he sounded more like a knight arduously standing by his broken mother.

"Please John Paul listen to me. You definitely need to go to Canada and reunite with your father. A treatment must already be available there; I'll meet you all later," I pleaded, trying to convince him of the irrationality of his plan. "No, Mom, I won't do that. I'll stay here. That way, I'll come to visit you until your release. I'll even find work to pay for my upkeep and you aren't going to make me change my mind." Obstinately, he insisted.

"J.P. you know as well as I do that it will be such a waste of time for you! The people who at first spoke to you said that it could take months before I even go to trial" I reminded him, hoping he would realize the futility of his idea. "Oh Mom, don't be silly please. I just can't and I won't leave France until we go together, okay?"

"Okay, okay." Momentarily I agreed with him. There was no need to contradict his good intentions now. Later when he was free, we could ultimately decide what was best, and in closing the subject now I told him. "Just remember that the Legal Aid lawyer believes that you will be liberated soon. At that time will talk about your plans. Okay?"

These intimate moments, even if short, kept John Paul and me in some way collected while we waited for the good results our lawyer had promised. The visits were extra special for me because from one week to the next my depleted batteries got recharged. Besides that, the stronger topic of our conversations necessarily was mutual concerns, bedecked by some of our daily experiences in prison.

Except that we never had enough time to go into depth on any subject. So we extended it in our letters. The existing vigilant censorship didn't intimidate us. John Paul and I had nothing to hide; everything about my offense was out in the open!

Going a few days back, January 28th Judith informed me that Martha and Steven arrived. Used to doing things efficiently they immediately hired a good lawyer for their sister, *Maitre* Thibault. The very same reputable and expensive lawyer J.P.' cellmates recommended was now Judith's attorney and because they came from abroad, *maitre* Thibault obtained special visiting rights for them. The D.A.'s office authorized visits for almost every day and for sessions longer than the usual assigned time.

Unable to keep her excitement after one of those visits, Judith gave me a scoop on the cause of her agitation. "Martha and Steve came today and brought me great news. Lydia got in touch with them. She has a plan to have me released. Obviously, it will cost some money, but my siblings are willing to pay to make it happen. Isn't this wonderful, Myriam?"

It sounded bizarre more than anything and truthfully I felt downhearted. Not because of me, it was because of my son. John Paul was unjustly detained and his fate hung in the hands of a state appointed lawyer while Judith, who was guilty, at least not in the magnitude that I was, had now the chance to be freed. I found the situation unfair and it gave me an uneasy feeling. The friend Judith was talking about was the woman who allegedly found the contact for the cocaine, and in my mind the one who gave us away.

In any event my antennas got instantly erected when Judith repeated some phrases the women told to her siblings, "I'm a good friend with *Monsieur* Clavier *le juge d'instruction.* He'll personally see that Judith is released on schedule, I promise." The woman's assertion was powerful; that man was the judge in charge of our case. I had the feeling she had something hidden under her sleeve and my gut feeling told me, "She's up to no good." And I trembled.

So far, Judith had not mentioned how her friend planed to obtain her release, nor the amount of money she had requested, but all seemed conceivable; no wonder her siblings had agreed to pay. Other than to me it sounded alarming; even more since I knew nothing about the French laws or the way their justice system worked. In any event my dislike for the women increased.

Yet I smothered the lot, simply because I didn't want to loose the chance however small, to obtain for John Paul the same help. So, directly I asked Judith, "Will you talk with your friend and see if she would intercede on my son's behalf too; bearing in mind that John Paul is truly innocent. You know this as well as I do, Judith!" I strongly emphasized.

I hated to have to appeal to that woman, but my son's freedom was more important than my likes or dislikes. I could be totally wrong and she could after all be a good person. Judith happy to act on my plea, a few days later told me, "My friend has agreed to use her influence to help your son too." At this point she also mentioned, "My siblings have paid her the money she asked. My release should happen any minute now." A couple of weeks went by, time in which Judith was not only visited by her siblings, but also by her friend. Evidently several times and the visits necessarily had to be authorized by the District Attorney.

Even with the load of worries on my mind, it was impossible to ignore the problems people around me had unless I wanted to be labeled as stuck-up. So I sometimes had to force myself to listen to other's confidences, especially my cellmates'. In a way I had done the same. Each knew about my offense. They first read it in the newspaper and later when asked, I confirmed the issues.

This particular day, both Danielle and Josee were called away from the cell, a visit from their lawyers perhaps, leaving Inge and I by ourselves. It wasn't that I encouraged her to talk. No, actually I would have preferred not to know anything too personal about them, but Inge chose this moment of privacy to share with me her concern. I had no other choice than to be a good listener.

"Myriam, I don't know if you are aware or not, but before my incarceration, my husband and I were respectable people. We came from Berlin to retire in Cannes, because thanks to the exchange rate, Gunter's small pension from Germany went further here in France than in our country. Unfortunately the situation changed, the exchange rate dropped and the money was no longer enough."

As she paused for a moment, I noticed her embarrassment and her eyes seemed shinier than usual, but she composed herself and continued, "Gunter developed a system of accessing money from other people's credit cards. The police arrested my husband for fraud." Tears poured freely down her cheeks now. Touched by her unhappiness, I reached out and held her hand in a sign of support.

"I wasn't involved in the offense, I swear to you Myriam. However, because I enjoyed in the proceeds, I was tried and brought to prison with him. I'll be released soon, but Gunter has to stay for eighteen more months. I don't know what will happen to me, once I'm out. I have no money, nor family!" She probably was past her sixties and was fearful for the uncertainty ahead. I honestly hoped the best for her, and audibly said, "Inge, you probably don't need to worry so much. Surely France or Germany will look after you until Gunter is out. They won't just leave you abandoned; you are a senior." I supposed that was all she needed to hear. By the time the others return, she was calm.

On another occasion it was Danielle, a short person with blond flat hair who had nothing attractive going for her. In my view, she even seemed to lack personality. Until one day she straightened me out on my ideas and told me how she happened to land at the *Maison d'Arret*. Otherwise, I would have never guessed, "I was the head accountant in this large firm in town; every day thousands of Francs went through my fingers, figuratively speaking because they were only numbers. You do understand, right?"

Not sure if I did or not, I just nodded and she continued talking, "For about four years I diverted some funds into my own account. One day I was discovered and ended up here. I only have six more months to serve of the three years I was given. Then, I'll be free. I plan to go to Bermuda and stay there. Woo!" She must have had a lot of nerve and a cool mind to accomplish the embezzlement. She probably had the money stashed away some place in Bermuda, where later she would happily enjoy the profits. She didn't say any of that, I just let my imagination have a run for it.

Now Josee, who I thought knew all the ins and outs of the prison system, because she was just a vivacious girl, I learned was not really like that. Apparently her husband and Josee, both, had been in and out of prison several times; their way of making a living was as common break and entry thieves. An occupation she wasn't a bit shy about, instead in conversations in the group, I heard her brag about it.

She loved to talk a lot about herself but also about other inmates, such as who faced murder charges and which ones were detained for trafficking and possession of drugs that supposedly was a large percentage. I believe my name was not part of her gossip, though I don't know why.

Judith and I often witnessed quarrels in the courtyard. The hitting, the scratching and hair yanking, while foul language was used, were all very real. Similar to scenes we see in the movies as paid spectators, but here, they were frightening. In these instances, male guards were called immediately to put a stop to the battle. The clashes involved the two predominant groups; these women when angered became dangerous; it was best not to side with either one.

At times the quietness of the night was broken by loud screams. It sounded, as if someone was being killed in one of the cells. In spite of everything and still trying to swim ashore, I took advantage of the Sundays' afternoon promenade to find some space for myself. Normally a quiet day in the courtyard, only a few inmates took this stroll. Here is where I met an interesting Italian woman, a little older than I, and very good-looking. At a younger age she must have been stunning.

My introduction to more stories continued with her. At first and still at a distance, I was intrigued by her dazzling looks. She seemed cultured and well educated. Perhaps because we had certain commonalities, a few Sundays after my arrival, she looked for my company. Her name was Monique du Mount Serrate, her mother tongue Italian, though she also spoke fluent French, Spanish and English; I believe she even had the command of more languages.

Her story was like a novel, interesting and absorbing. Monique had been married to an Italian Count; or so she said. Through this marriage she had luxury, money, palaces, servants, but no children. Madame du Mount Serrate left her husband and all the comforts she had with him behind, when she met and fell in love with a younger man. It was not until much later that she found out he was a famous bank robber who even had murder charges on his record and was wanted by the police in several countries throughout Europe.

Discovering this truth about her lover didn't stop her infatuation. Monique kept the relationship going even after he was caught and both were sent to prison. According to her story, she was never involved in any of his delinquent life but just the same, she ended up arrested. On the date of their trial, accomplices of the gangster set-up an ambush on the way to the Court and he was able to escape but Monique was left behind.

She implied that five years had gone by since the day of her arrest and that the case was still open, because her lover, even now, was on the run. I can't vouch for the truth of her tale or for her innocence, but her stories were a welcome change of pace in my captive life. Stillness equaled monotony, plus my added worries logically could easily prompt me into a depression mode; a variation in tone was always welcome.

February brought something remarkable. The first week of the month I received a letter from Mr. Andrew Covet, the Canadian vice-consul in Marseilles, with a copy sent to John Paul. I was beside myself with the news.

February 2, 1986

> *Dear Mrs. Arthur, your husband has recently contacted this consulate to inform us that he will soon be sending a large amount of money. He has ordered us, to instruct you to retain a reputable lawyer for your defense. He also strongly recommends that no money should be spared to obtain John Paul's prompt release. Your husband and this office will be in constant communication; it appears that for the moment it is Mr. Arthur's best way to obtain news from both you and your son. We will inform you the minute the check is in our hands. In the mean time we will be pleased to remain at your service, sincerely yours, etc.*

John surely had received my letter and had included me in his favorable disposition. His decision gave me a clearer view of the man he really was! My morale was boosted, yet I realized my husband had to incur a lot of difficulties to get hold of the money he intended to send; all our holdings were back in Bolivia. John likely had to resort to his parents and asked them for a loan, but the letter could not have come at better time.

The Legal Aid lawyer, who promised positive results for John Paul, had not yet visited him, nor come back to see me after her first appearance. Even before I got the letter from the consulate, I started to wonder if she had the knowledge or if she had any interest in our case. All was just too preposterous, our needs had not changed; we required a diligent lawyer not a sleeping beauty. But now with excellent news I could take another course of action.

In a sense, her lack of concern liberated me from any commitment I might have had with her. John's specific instructions to the Consul cleared the way. "Retain a good lawyer to obtain John Paul's prompt release." I had to find and hire a good attorney; too much was at risk for our son if I waited any longer. Meticulously and without delay I went over the list of the salaried attorneys, hopping one, English or Spanish speaking would vividly grasp my attention!

No such luck, the names bore no suggestions, John Paul, aware of his Dad' letter, brought *Maitre* Thibault's name back to the table. The man spoke English all right, but was already retained by Judith. J. P. then suggested, "Mom you should ask for the advice of the Consulate." This was perfect input, considering I was becoming frantic. Unfortunately all I got from that office was another list of lawyers, with the usual "we can't get involved" stuff.

Surely some inmates had to know of a good lawyer. I checked around still with no luck. Looking for a needle in a haystack would have been easier; no one had ever needed a lawyer with the qualifications I was seeking. Monique suggested, "*Maitre* Alain Portiere is my lawyer and he is excellent. I have never spoken English with him but I believe he does. You'll have to ask him yourself," she said, confident her referral would meet my criteria.

"Portiere is getting my case open and tried with my lover in absentia. He's worked hard to have it done. Otherwise I could easily rot in prison; the judge's intention was to wait until the police caught him. He has done wonders for me." Monique kept talking about Portiere with enthusiasm, exactly what I needed to hear, which helped me decide. "You can check with other girls, they'll tell you the same. He has a good reputation among the inmate population, Portiere gets things done." Very much at ease with her suggestion she smiled and added, "I wish you good luck, Myriam."

A sound referral, yet I had to be sure. John Paul had left the choice entirely in my hands saying, "Now that my father is backing you up financially, Mom, you need to have the best lawyer for your defense." I wanted just that, but primarily to expedite my son's liberation and since *Maitre* Portiere seemed to have a perfect reputation, I opted for him. Quickly I wrote to the lawyer requesting his services.

I didn't have to wait long for his response. Two days later *Maitre* Portiere came to see me. Impressed by his quick reply, I paid no heed to Elizabeth's interim visit to J.P. She had showed up the day before, but after two weeks of silence, I felt more than exonerated from her services.

The lawyer's features were somewhat familiar. I had seen him not too long ago; I was on my way to my French classes and he was talking to Sylvie, who was doing her cleaning chores in the hallway, downstairs. His peppery hair was what had caught my attention, almost all grey, unusual for a man of his age, perhaps no older than forty or forty-five. At a much closer range now I could see Maitre Portiere had a distinct look, was well-built, moderate height and in general had an attractive appearance.

As he started to talk, I noticed his command of the English language was not what I had expected it to be! It came with a very heavy French accent; the inflection hindered my understanding. Time after time, I had to ask him to repeat phrases but his diligence and the outstanding referral from Dominique made me overlook the rest. On the other hand, he didn't seem to have any trouble understanding me. He absorbed everything I said, taking notes, but most of the time just listening.

In detail I went over our arrest, my crime, the plot and my motive. I made sure he was well aware John Paul had no part in my crime, "Maitre Portiere, it's very important you understand my son had no part in my offense. The reason why John Paul was with me might sound very foolish, but it's the truth! I'll explain it to you if I may?" I paused, the sobbing was about to start, but I managed to control myself.

"Originally my plan was to go to Barcelona by plane. Unfortunately I did not book the reservation ahead and upon my arrival in Nice, I found all the flights were sold out. My rendez-vous to deliver the drug was at 5 pm. December 31; we arrived in France the 29, I hardly had any time left." *Maitre* Portiere didn't say a word; he just silently listened and stared at me.

Very uncomfortable, my mouth was dry but I continued, "I decided to rent a car instead. Unwisely I asked my son to drive me to Spain. John Paul only knew I was going to Barcelona to see a friend, a doctor, who aware of his illness was going to give us a referral letter for a specialist in Paris. My son is infected with AIDS and he didn't know I carried in my suitcase 700g of cocaine."

I was almost ready to break down, but I remained strong for a while longer, "My son's imprisonment is a big mistake. John Paul is here only because he happened to be with me at the moment of my arrest. He had nothing to do with my crime." The attorney still looked at me with inquisitive eyes. I didn't know if he was trying to read the veracity of my words or his prolonged silence meant he had not understood a word I said? What ever it was, I felt it was an invitation for me to continue and so I did, "My need for an attorney more than anything is to clarify this mistake."

Maitre Portiere finally spoke, but what he said was unbeliev-able. Actually I was stunned by his words. "Madame Arthur, you risk a very harsh sentence. Possibly a twelve to fifteen years of imprisonment."

Baffled by his statement I asked myself, why anyone would want to give such a harsh sentence to a desperate mother. A sentence such as the one *Maitre* Portiere mentioned, was surely given to people involved in intense trafficking, where millions of dollars were made. My case could not possibly be treated as such; at least that much I learned from other inmate's experiences, as well as from what John Paul had found out from his side.

Probably he was just trying to scare me to increase his fees, or I misunderstood everything he said because of his accent, I thought. I didn't have chance to ask him directly because his next words overshadowed his previous statement. "On the other hand, your son will be out of here in no time." This announcement was enough for me! To have the reassurance of this reputable lawyer that John Paul's release was unquestionable! It was the answer I was waiting to hear. The rest, though it was tough it did not matter that much.

The session with *Maitre* Portiere ended and as he got up ready to depart, he handed me a piece of paper where the amount of forty-five thousand Francs was written; supposedly the fee to take over our defense. He could have written one million francs; it would not have made any difference!

First because of his uplifting words, "There won't be any problem in clearing your son." Secondly, because I had no idea what the conversion of that amount into dollars represented and I didn't ask. What is more, in my view I thought he was even trying to make things easier for me, when he suggested, "Mrs. Arthur, you may pay in installments if you wish." Eager to get John Paul out of prison, I accepted. He then shook my hand and left.

The same day in the evening, I wrote to my son, giving him the news about *Maitre* Portiere, the new lawyer I hired, plus the details of the interview and his fees.

Feb. 5th

How are you Mamita linda?

Today Elizabeth came to see me. She apologized for not coming before, and explained that she was not able to do anything yet. Supposedly because the District Attorney is gathering more information on us, like checking with Interpol to find out if we have had previous criminal records in our background. I had to laugh and told her, "It will be great if they hurry up, because we don't have any unlawful matters behind us, and perhaps then things will start moving." She was here only for a few minutes; will be back as soon as there is a fixed date for the interrogatory sessions.

That is all I can say about her; nothing exciting as you can see. Except that just now I've been notified that Dad has sent some money through the Consulate for canteen expenditures. I still have close to 1,200.00 Francs left from the money you transferred to my account. So, right now, I don't need any. It will be best if it's all deposited into yours; I'm almost certain you hardly have any left. Be serious Mom, you need it to subsidize some of the daily necessities available through the canteen. This time, Mom, you better listen to me and write to the Consulate to this effect, or I will.

Did I tell you about my French teacher? His name is Sylvan and he is an awesome guy. I have often talked about you, with him. He knows Claudette and has offered to hand over to your teacher some books I found in the library, good ones. I've read them myself. You'll like them.

Guess what? He is aware I am an artist and wants me to paint a fresco in the classroom. He only needs the final okay from the warden, to let me start. It will be my work. Thanks to my talent, I'm becoming very popular around this wonderful Jet Set milieu. Seriously though, I believe most people here, are starting to appreciate us, probably because we show that we are caring people.

Do you realize Mom that God has created all human creatures with the power of love, but only a few are fortunate enough to grasp it. The rest, don't even know that the Son of God died because of his infinite love for humanity. It's sad to find people who still don't want to accept this reality.

Mom, as much as I love writing to you, right now I must say good night; I'm falling sleep.

Love you, J.P.

February 6th

Hello Mother,

Had I known yesterday, when Elizabeth came, that you hired Maitre Portiere as our new counselor, I would have mentioned that to her. I supposed you will deal with her the next time she goes around to see you.

In regards to Maître Portiere, I didn't know what to make out of what he told you, so in doubt I checked with people here. I realized their credibility is not the best, but in prison matters, I believe they have a lot of experience and can give sound advice.

About the fifteen years sentence he hung over your head; they think the same as you, and I, that he has exaggerated to justify his fee. I trust their input. First, because they are French, have been long enough in prison, have seen an adequate amount of stuff around here and heard of sufficient cases, which gives them certain amount of knowledge in topics such as this.

About if he is good? Yes, he is. In regards to the forty-five thousand Francs he is charging, in their view the price is high. According to them, fifteen thousand Francs for each of us is enough. It's what any other good lawyer charges and in more complicated cases than ours. They have advised me to tell you that lawyers are money hungry; when they smell a good profit they take advantage.

To obtain a better price, you need to bargain with him. Apparently it is a common practice around here. Once he agrees, because he will, you have to stipulate that you will pay him in accordance to the time and effort he puts into our case. Make sure that the Consulate is aware of this and that any payments to him should only be made under your written authorization.

I have to go now, its bedtime. Enclose, you will find some of my drawings. I hope they'll cheer you up. Love, J.P.

February 7th

Dear Mom,

Did you get my last letter? I hope so; it had information about lawyers and fees. Please Mother, I don't want to hear you say ever again that you are selfish because you feel comforted by having me near you. Once and for all, I want you to know that I wouldn't want to be in any other place in the world.

In a lighter mode, I'll tell you about Charlie one of my roommates. I think I told you about him already; he is a gem. He always is offering me all kinds of treats. When his family comes to visit him, he even sends my clothes along with his, to have them washed. Did you know this could be done? Not us of course, we don't have any family around. Anyway it's great, lately I never lack clean and fresh clothes and I love it because I don't have to do it myself anymore. In exchange, I draw some portraits of his family. This place wouldn't be too bad if only the doors weren't locked from the outside.

From what you tell me, your roommates are good too, and going to classes keeps your mind occupied. Soon we will learn directly from Mr. District Attorney on what plans he has.

Love you Mom, J.P.

February 8th.

My dear Mom,

I really don't understand what is happening with the internal mail service. It's not that the censuring has to go to Paris and back, who knows, maybe it does; Paris is only a joke Mom. (Note: To the person who censures the letters. Please, have a heart. Being behind bars is hard enough; not receiving our correspondence makes it even more difficult. Thank you).

I've some news to give you, Mom. The more I talked with the guys on what I know about our case, the more they've reassured me that I should be out of this place in a cinch. They actually don't see any reason for my detention. So with that, Maitre Portiere is right. In your case however, they say you'll have a trial first, but they don't think your sentence will be too harsh. No more than eighteen months. In this, as you can see, he is totally wrong!

Another possibility is that right after the trial; you could be deported; a fine or a tax on the quantity of the imported drug will be set. I'm sure father will do his best to obtain the money when the time comes. I'll certainly pray this will be the solution. I can't stand the possibility that you might spend time in prison.

Someone from another group told me that most attorneys are money hungry and play strange tricks on their clients. Supposedly, here in France, it isn't like in America where lawyers work entirely on their client's behalf.

About myself, so that you know, I'm following your instructions. Every week, I make sure to include in my order from the canteen, fresh fruit, especially lemons and oranges, yogurt, milk, cheese, sardines; that healthy staff you wanted me to eat. Did you know that we could even order and pay for special dishes? It would be good to have fish in my diet once in a while.

By the time you receive this letter one more of our lovely visits will have gone by. It's a lot nicer when I get to talk to you in person; it breaks the monotony. Writing is okay too, a necessity for us! Give my regards to Judith and your roommates.

All my love for you, Mom, J. P.

Feb. 9th.

Dearest Mother,

Once again it's Sunday, and even though I'm still filled with the joy of our reunion last Thursday, it seems to be fading away. I'm already looking forward to the next one. I don't see why the system doesn't make these visits an every day event and call it a rehabilitation program. Every one could benefit from it, even the guards.

Now, I can't hold it any longer. I have to tell you! Friday, I received news from Dad, and Patrick. From the dates; seems that the District Attorney's censoring ringer had them, for over fourteen days.

Supposedly these letters were the second ones they had written. I wonder if the first set, is still somewhere in their archives covered with spider webs and lost for good. I understand father and Patrick, wrote to you, too. The way the censoring works, who knows, you might have received them already, or are you still in suspense? Just in case, I'll share with you the major points in their letters.

Father has decided to stay in Canada, and he is looking for work in Vancouver and Calgary.

Dad wants a new start for the family...and plans to sell all that we own back in Bolivia. Do you realize Mom? When Dad was making this decision, I was thinking exactly the same. I must have extra sensory perception (ESP) you always said I had it. You knew, I could read your thoughts almost to the dot, remember? I supposed later I must have lost it, because, although I sensed something wasn't quite right in our trip to France, I just couldn't pin down what it was

Going back to Dad's letter, hold on tight Mom, this might shake you up a bit more. It seems that every one of our friends in Bolivia is aware of what happened to us here in France, our detention was printed in a newspaper from Santa Cruz. Rudy called Dad; he had read the article, and concerned about us offered his assistance. He assured Dad, that he, his wife, and many others will look after Grandmother, while our situation is resolved.

In Canada, Uncle Ken is the only one who knows. Dad doesn't want his parents to know. He thinks it would be too hard on them and finds no need to give them such bad news. My little brother also knows. He wrote, saying that neither he nor Dad hold any judgment against you. Patrick explained in a few words that father's reason for not returning to Bolivia is because he fears other

friends and relatives might not be as understand-
ing as Rudy was.

*Dad won't mention anything about the article
in the newspaper to you, since he doesn't want
to put one more concern over your shoulders. If
I bring it up now, it's because I feel that sooner
or later you'll find out; and its best you learn it
from me.*

*My feeling goes to Dad; I don't blame him for
this decision. You know he can't stand gossip, least
if his family is the reason of the scandal. Besides,
can you imagine the shock all this must have been
for him? Sorry Mom, try not to worry too much.
We should leave everything in the Lord's hands.
I'm sure He'll look after us. Anyway, it was great
to receive their letters. I hope you got yours as
well. Let me know.*

*I'm praying this letter doesn't take forever to
reach you. It's lengthy, and risks collecting some
dust at le Juge's censoring department, but by
now all the staff must be bored with us having to
read our letters every day with nothing new!*

Love you, J.P.

Just before my son received the letters from his Dad and
Patrick, our morale was down; at least, mine was. With no family
or friends close by, the disconnection was hard. The vice-consul's
missive helped but it was not the same. Completely cut off from

the outside world, my son's proximity was a great blessing and selfishly I believed he was near to help me walk through this part of my detainment, while his release was in the works!

My son's guess was right. I had not received any letters, but now thanks to his intuitive concern, I got the news. It freed my mind a little. I had feared my husband's silence meant he had no desire to have any further contact with me. Evidently I was wrong, what is more I had no reason to battle John's decision to relocate the family permanently to Canada. In reality, I found his choice opportune and right. I had no desire to return to my country either, being that our situation was out in the open. It would represent a bombshell to my pride, which I still had.

February 11[th.] I got the letters, one posted in Canada, the other from Bolivia. The envelopes were opened and placed inside a large manila cover; the dissecting group from the D.A.'s office naturally read the news before I did. As I started to re-open the one from Canada, I was petrified. Part of me wanted to engulf its contents at once, but afraid to find out all that my husband had to say, I hesitated. Finally with trembling hands, I opened the envelope and there it was a long letter from my husband, a shorter one from Patrick.

Oh my God, I could not believe it! My heart seemed ready to explode with angst as I read John's letter and felt his pain. It was not what I had expected. My husband could not have been more shocked after he received my confession, but he didn't judge me, condemn or condone me. He was just as sad. If until then I had not realized the magnitude of his love, any doubts were immediately erased. It was the guilt I carried that made feel as a despicable worm, not any of his words!

From my husband's letter, I learned that John first found out of our predicament through a telephone call from Wayne, Judith's oldest brother. He had called from the United States, giving him the bad news of our mishap after Judith's family was notified by her husband. John didn't know him that well and at first thought it was a prank. Wayne was a man of a few words, the less he said the better he felt.

All John knew was that I went to France on business, but Wayne made him aware that we were incarcerated for drug trafficking. Was I lying then, when I told him, I was going to Nice to introduce the splendid Bolivian artisan's crafts in the French Market? Was that a fabricated story; was John Paul to blame?

Apparently all those questions went through my husband's mind. He was heartbroken, and had no idea what was going on, but realized that even if I was the one responsible, he could not ever stop loving me. Even so he didn't condone what I had done, yet neither was he closing the door down on me. John in his noble heart allowed himself to think that I must have had a very compelling reason to do what I did.

Following the incoherent conversation with Wayne, still unable to grasp this information, he contacted the Canadian authorities in Paris. Transferred to the Canadian Consulate in Marseilles, office in charge for all Southern France, John talked to the vice-consul. Who after he listened to my husband's concern, "I just learned that my wife Myriam Arthur and my son John Paul are in some kind of trouble with the law, detained somewhere in the South of France. Will you be so kind to find out all you can about this situation?" The vice-consul promised to do so.

Later through a second phone call, John was filled in; the prison's social assistants had filled in some of the blanks. My husband had to accept the accuracy of Wayne's information and gently break the bad news to my mother and sister. Vicky, immediately took the first flight available to Cochabamba to be by my Mom's side, hoping the damage of the news on her health, would not be irreversible.

The whole lot was more like a nightmare for my husband, who until then was having a grand time visiting his parents. In addition a few days down the road when John was just barely recovering from the reports of our incarceration, he received my letter and my husband had to bear the pain of learning our son had AIDS.

My heart went out to him. All the grief I caused and the worst was that all had been for nothing. The disease was still on its destructive path and we were in prison.

After my heart had settled a bit, I read Patrick's letter. My precious son, who in all his young life had my love and protection, of course his Dad's too, suddenly was hit by the horrific news of our arrest! His reaction was also incredibly non-judgmental. Instead, cheerfully he tried to comfort me. Perhaps because he was too young to grasp the seriousness of my fault, he only saw the fact that his brother needed my help, the rest was irrelevant.

Patrick always had showed such a tremendous amount of love and wisdom. What caressed me the most of his letter were his phrases, "Mom, don't worry, I love you just the same, no matter what. Now, we need to get you and J.P. back with us; my brother has to get better!"

In the last while, Patrick had seen the worst of our life style, the drinking and smoking. He reproached us, but only with loving words. Patrick's goal was to make us realize the harm we were doing to ourselves with our excess life style and presently he was faced yet with this new quandary. Not a nice scenario for Patrick, he was barely fifteen years old and cruelly all the security he once had was destroyed by a simple telephone call and a letter; his childhood was lost and Patrick became a man.

My mother's letter was a different story, she was heartbroken, but because of the love she had for me, Mom could not see that I could do any wrong, I was her baby. Besides, the situation was too complicated for her to understand a whole lot, who would anyway? So, Mother blamed it all, on Judith.

As I finished reading the letters, I should have been freed from my anguish of being abandoned by my family. In a sense I was, but the concern and remorse remained, but took another dimension. Through my life I had taken them for granted and only now I realized the horrendous aftermath I had left behind me.

Feb 12th

Dear Mom,

I just finished reading my mail. It troubles and saddens me to learn the effect that Dad's and Patrick's letters had on you. If they would have rejected you, cursed you, or been angry with you, I could understand your distress, or embarrassment, if you want to call it that way. Then, you might have had a good reason to feel bad, but they didn't. Instead, both of them have shown you only their love and understanding. Also Grandma, even if she was a bit mixed-up. It's now time to stop all this nonsense, Mom!

As a matter of fact, I've a lot of respect for Dad. It's admirable in the way he reacted to the whole situation! About the news reaching Bolivia, it doesn't really matter Mom; because the people, who sincerely care for us, wouldn't allow the bond of friendship of an entire lifetime to be destroyed just because we are in prison.

Truthfully Mom, don't you find it's better for us not to return to Bolivia, as father wants and I agree with him. I'm sorry to have to say this to you, but things over there weren't right anymore. I believe the country was in total decadence, because of the corruption. Then, there were those selfish and envious people around us, who pretended to be friends, I can almost see their satisfaction the moment they hear about our problem. Certainly not the true friends, who are people like us; who would be able to recognize that no one is exempt from making mistakes.

We have always been a courageous family, and we aren't going to lose our courage now, are we, Mother? On the contrary, this is a time we need to be strong and show to everyone that we'll be able to continue on with our lives, once this is over. I'm glad though, that it will be in a new frontier. In Canada, the country we should have never left and where I'm sure we will still have a life full of good fortune.

So please Mother, put aside all those thoughts, because our destiny has just begun. Remember that God has ways to show us what He really wants from us. Mom, promise me, that you won't worry anymore. Have peace in your mind and heart. You thought that what you were doing was right, only out of the love you had for me.

I love you J. P.

RECONNECTING WITH CHRIST

In this troublesome stage, it is when I first met Rev. Fray Regis, the Catholic Chaplain at the precinct. The minute I learned inmates could have the priest's weekly visits, I requested to be put on the list, but the red tape delayed this privilege for almost three weeks.

After, I saw Fray Regis every Friday. He came into my life as a priest, but I also found in him a friend and his visits helped me a lot. With him I could openly talk about what troubled me the most: my son's ailing condition. In addition I confessed my sins too; even though it was not easy to humbly summarize all that I had done wrong. Undoubtedly he saw my remorse and in the name of our Lord, he absolved all my transgressions.

I wished it had been that simple for me. It didn't work that way. Even as sincerely remorseful as I was, stubbornly I felt unworthy of God's pardon, or from anyone's forgiveness for that matter. My guilt was too imbedded, it was difficult to accept the Lord's blessed forgiveness and be at peace with myself.

Father Regis kept coming back to help rebuild my faith. He patiently refreshed my memory on things I had learned in the past. Such as that our Father in heaven because of His infinite love for us, had sacrificed his only Son, so that my sins may be forgiven.

The priest admonished me, "Myriam, you must learn to accept the designs the Lord has for you." His words had a profound impact on my soul, but my personal wounds still didn't' allow me to understand. My heart was hardened to the Word, everything seemed the same as when I had lost my father, so I asked the priest, "Why God, as the loving Father he supposedly is, would allow my son's illness, his incarceration and even my own to happen? What is the purpose of all that has happened to us, if it only causes so much pain?"

With my thoughts fixed on my circumstances, I proceeded, "In my understanding, love implies protecting your children from any harm or suffering; it is beyond my human comprehension of any other way that love can be shown. So don't tell me that God's design for us was this?" Adamantly I questioned him.

Fray Regis, unperturbed by my rhetoric said, "Myriam, you have much yet to learn. You need to read the Bible to understand more about the Word! Soon it will come to you. He reached into his briefcase and handed me a Bible. This book will enlighten you on the Lord's Word. It will give you the strength you will need to face human justice, which is not as understanding or forgiving."

I had no qualms about his advice. I would read the Holy Bible from beginning to end, something, I had never done before. Rev. Fray Regis became another source of moral support for both John Paul and myself. He made himself available for my son too. His visits, plus the love shown by my family even after they learned what I had done, were very comforting.

Feb. 13th

Dear Mom,

I hope you are calmer now and able to see things from a brighter perspective. Just for example, look at the strength that God gave a mi abuelita, to help her walk through this troublesome time. Also the moral support that friends and relatives are giving to Dad and her. Then there is also father's wonderful idea to send for Grandmother so that we would care for her when we are all in Canada. I believe we are truly blessed. We have God's love, my Dad's and Patrick's. In my view this experience has united us more, made us better people. Father hasn't judged or questioned me about my illness. So you see, you need to keep positive and strong.

Lets talk about something else now, I heard very good things today; that inmates are able to earn yearly remissions on their sentence, three months for good conduct, three more months if you complete successfully the French course at school. And there might be another one yet, elections are coming up soon and sometimes politicians grant complete remissions to special cases.

There you are, with this news, I believe that neither you nor Judith will be here for long. So, keep a smile on your face. We all love you and that is what really counts. My new playmates think very dearly of you, too.

Love you, J.P.

P.S. Because of my resent move, I've lost connection with Rev. Fray Regis. No one seems to know when he will come around to this area. If you see him, please let him know about my change of residence. Perhaps, he can make it happen faster from his end.

Feb 17th

Dearest Mother,

(Note)I am addressing this note to the person in charge of censoring our mail. First, I wish you a good day, and secondly, I must give you many thanks for handing my letters over to my mother without delay.)

Mom, I know that this is not the best place to spend your wedding anniversary, twenty-six years right? It doesn't matter. It's still a great date to celebrate. I hope you received my humble creations, Ha-ha. I sent them a few days ago as a present.

Today was a day filled with excitement and oh how I wish everyday was the same. First in the morning we had our weekly visit, completed in the evening when I received the mail and got two Valentines cards, one from Dad and the other from Patrick.

For a change, the mail arrived right on time and brought us some joy. Yes I know, a little bird whispered in my ear that there was a large envelope for you too. So hopefully you will be able to forget your sorrows, at least for a while.

As for me it went beyond, my morale was lifted sky-high, all because of the love Dad and my little brother expressed in their cards. The many great things they said about me, made my head swell up with pride. I don't think anyone around here will be able to put up with me any more at least for a while. Ha, ha.

There was something else, yesterday while at the promenade, some guys from another group I met, insisted I could speed my way out of this place by asking our lawyer to apply for a conditional release.

They even offered to find a job for me through their friends outside; its one of the requirements for this type of release. The other is to have a place to reside. Perhaps I could stay at Judith's house. At first, I wasn't too enthused with the idea, thinking it might represent another expense for father, but it would be a different story if I have the certainty of a job.

I could pay for my own keep, and I would still be able to visit you. Better yet, I'll be well equipped to mobilize the lawyers on your behalf. The "Prefecture" is the office that provides working permits to foreigners for two months and up to five years. In the end, it would be great if I could stay in France, until you are released. It's something worthwhile looking for.

I believe I have now depleted my repertoire, but certainly I want to wish you a good night and tell you that I love you. J. P.

Feb. 18th

Dear Mom.

No, I'm not sick. Actually I'm feeling pretty good. Lately I'm finding great encouragement in my art. It seems as if the Muse that is inspiring me is trying to make up for the rest of the losses in my life. Truthfully, I'm creating beautiful pieces. In the past week I worked on a couple of portraits I made of Grandpa and Grandma. I'm very pleased; you'll have them in the next mail.

Because of the recent changes happening around here, I've lost Charlie's helping hand with my laundry, most upsetting. I've no other choice now than to wash and dry my clothes in this cubicle. No sweat, it gets done.

Thursdays are definitely the best day of the week for me. Yesterday after our visit, the rest of my day went by quickly. I insist we should have these visits every day.

I was almost forgetting, yesterday Josee's husband introduced himself and told me, "Your mother made a dress for my wife. She was wearing

it today and even through the glass at the parloir
I could appreciate it was beautiful. Josse was very
happy." From his description, I could almost see
it. I know your talent. What I can't imagine is
how did you managed to sew a dress entirely by
hand. You are amazing Mom

Then Sylvan completed my day; he has asked
me to do the drawings for the prison's newspaper,
and guess what? I'm going to be paid for it. The
money part will be good to have, but better yet will
be the daily showers. I won't stink so much any
more. He hasn't forgotten about the fresco for our
classroom. He is still trying to obtain the money
for the materials, but administration it's taking
forever to come up with it. Thankfully I will be
doing something else in the meantime.

But our teacher is eternally re-organizing
the student's habitat; and we are going through
another change. To make the move more pleasant, he wants us to put in writing our choice as to
whom we would like to have for roommates.

My choice was for anyone, except the Yugoslav.
You probably are asking yourself, "What happened, you used to like that guy; wasn't he the one
who was an intellectual type?" He was Mom, but
he turned out to be a moody person and very dis-
trustful of others.

He kept saying that some of the cubicles where we have our visits on Thursdays are wired to the head office. According to him, there is a device set to capture everything said in these intimate conversations. Since, I have some negative moments myself, I didn't think I needed this type of atmosphere around me.

Guess what? Almost everyone that goes to the French classes has requested to have me as their roommate. It makes me feel good, to be shown this appreciation, even in this setting. In all honesty and without any arrogance I can say that we are a very special family. As far back as I can remember we always extended our hands to help others. God is showing us the good returns now, even in prison. J. P.

Feb. 20th

Dear Mom, Did you see the snowstorm last night? The promenade was not mandatory today, it was too cold and too much snow accumulated in the courtyard. I went out anyway. I just can't be locked up for twenty-four hours without fresh air and some breathing space for myself.

About the changes, I understand a young Italian chap will be moved to our cell by tomorrow. Apparently he is just as popular as I am. I don't exactly know what his problem is, but he has been confined for the past five years without a trial. I have talked to him before; he seems to know from A to Z about the judicial system and what one can expect. According to him, our case is a piece of cake compared with other drug offenses.

Per example, right now, more than thirty inmates are being questioned at the Court of Grasse. They were involved in the importation and trafficking of hundreds if not thousands of kilos of heroin from Morocco. It seems that the trafficking was going on for at least four years. The District Attorney in this case, is demanding a 12-20 year sentence for the ringleaders, much less for the rest. I believe you know a couple of the girls involved in it, Sylvie and Corinne, the two girls who serve the meals, but there are more.

By the way, have you seen our lawyers lately? I haven't. I hope they show up soon. I'd like to find out when our first cross-examination will take place. I'm starting to get very impatient, as if it would make any difference. Still, I would love to have once and for all a good discussion with our dear Judge d'Instruction and straighten up his ideas!

About the conditional release, I mentioned before, I've changed my mind. I will not apply for it anymore. It wasn't such a good idea anyway.

I learned the friends, who were going to help me find work, happened to be quite involved with the underworld. I don't want to give any reason to the District Attorney to think I relate with people in that milieu. I'll just sit tight and patiently wait for the lawyers do their work.

Sleepy time now, but every night before I go to sleep, I thank God for delivering us from something worse and for keeping our family together through this difficult time and lately I mostly pray that He keeps you healthy. Love J. P.

Vendredi, Fevrier 22

Ma Mere,

Everybody be prepared, this is a long letter. It's divided into parts so I'll not forget anything.

1st - I've the feeling you are still lost with your directions; you really don't have a clue where the south might be. I'll help you find your bearings, if you face the big wall of the court that is south. Your left arm will be pointing east, and your right, west; as soon as you have these facts straight, you'll be able to see me soon.

Yes, I'm that close to you. Every day around 4.30 pm., I'll be on the look out for you from the shower window. At that time you must check for me too, from the window you girls have in the hall, the one between your cell and the staircase. Okay?

2ⁿᵈ- I received another letter from Dad and Patrick, dated February 10th. They seemed more relaxed after the vice-consul informed them about my health. Dad has requested him, to regularly check with the social assistant on this. They know now we are both fine.

You likely received similar letters, but just in case I am quoting a few important parts; Dad insists we need to have a good lawyer for our defense, but also sees the importance of keeping Elizabeth, so as per his instructions through the Consulate he has authorized the expenditure for her too.

Dad has financed the money for the retaining fees and feels confident the house we have under construction, will sell in time to pay for both lawyers. With so many things in his hands, father hasn't given one hundred percent of his time to search for a job. Besides, he wants to be accessible for any contingencies, or for anything we might need.

Patrick is coping well with the changes. He is in school and has many friends, mainly girls, all crazy over his Spanish accent. He's happy to be in Canada, and hopes we'll soon join them. Then, the whole family will be together again. Our letters seemed to take almost two weeks to arrive to their destination. If there is anything urgent we need to transmit, Dad suggests we do it through the Consulate.

3rd - I'm enclosing my latest art creation, which by the way makes me very proud. Once I'm free I'd like to exhibit all I've done here. In the meantime, it makes me happy to have you as my best art critic. I hope you'll enjoy it, as much as I did.

I'm done with numbering. Now I want to ask you something special. Please stop blaming yourself for this situation, okay. It's no one's fault what happened and it's a waste of time to keep thinking about the past. There is nothing we can do to change it and in my view to dwell about it is the worst sin we can perpetrate against ourselves. So please stop!

If you are still having those horrible headaches, please see the doctor. I believe at your side, the same as here they have something like a clinic set up, where every two weeks or so a doctor comes around and fixes the major problems. Make sure you get an appointment.

It's now time to say good night. I hope this big package gets to you for the weekend. The drawing was meant to be my present for your wedding anniversary; sorry it's a few days late.

Love J. P.

Feb. 25th

Dear Mom,

Sylvan finally got the materials for the fresco in our classroom. He thinks I should be able to start the project next week and has asked me to show him the sketch I prepared.

I'll explain what I drew: In the background the Canadian Rocky Mountains partly covered with snow, at the front two log cabins stand next to a stream of rippled crystal water; to give this effect I plan to combine blue and white colors, stroked fast and if needed, I can always add some more white. A dirt road trails into the mountain surrounded by a thick forest of spruce and pine trees. Too bad, you can't come to see it, but I'm sure you can follow my explanation, right? My teacher was pleased!

Then this afternoon, to give us a break instead of having the regular French class, he decided we would watch Gandhi's life on video. It is the second time I have seen this film, but still brought tears to my eyes. It probably sounds odd, but there is something therapeutic about tears, at least for me. After I shed them, I feel as if my burdens are lifted away. How great must be the love that God has for us that has even provided such a complex and perfect mechanism; I can only stand in awe at His marvelous wonders.

Now without fibs Mom; how are you feeling? I'm worried about the headaches you're having. I wish you would take your health more seriously. Have a doctor check this problem. It could be nothing, as you say, but better be on the safe side. (Note, I ask the person, who is censoring this letter to make sure a doctor sees my mother. Thank you).

This week, I must declare, I went beyond my means in my order from the canteen. I was tired of the gloomy look of my sketches. I wanted the new character I've created for you to keep you company, to be a happy little guy. He required a more colorful wardrobe to dress up when he goes to visit you. I now have all the colored pencils I need

My escape from this place is my drawings. Without this gift and the inspiration that God has given me, I'd probably just vegetate like the rest around me do. I'm relieved to know that you occupy your time with your classes, as long as you don't forget you have a son at this side, okay.

I love you, J. P.

P.S. I almost forgot to tell you, Charlie is back as my roommate. Hurray! I don't have to worry about laundering my clothes again. I was starting to lose weight with the work out. Ha-ha.

Mardi, Février 26

Ma chère Maman,

Did you receive Dad's first letter? Probably not, who knows you might still get it. It surprised me to receive mine, after such a long time. Just in case I'll tell you all about the one I received.

Father blames himself for everything seeing that he was unable to notice all the stress you carried alone. He realizes his mistakes, not taking a more effective part in the decision-making on the partnership and our own financial estate of our affairs for one. Dad has promised himself, not to let that happen ever again. I also sensed his hurt; you hadn't told him anything.

That is just it Mom, you never let anyone of us know if something serious affected our lives and in the midst of that mess, I brought you my own jam; I asked you to keep my secret from Dad. I'm not sure what I was thinking. Had I know the reality of our situation; honestly, I don't know what I would have done? I'm at fault too; I unloaded so much on you!

Anyhow, I believe Rose knew more about our internal affairs than the rest of us. Please don't take this as a criticism. I'm glad that at least you had someone to confide in, as I confided in you. Nothing will ever make me change the way I feel towards you. I'm proud to be your son and I'm sure that my father and brother have the same appreciation for you. Thankfully Dad was able to take immediate control of the situation.

In this letter, the same as his last, the, he announced his decision to stay in Canada permanently, and my brother backs him up one hundred per cent. Patrick is already attending school; the same level as in Bolivia. Took some tests and in most of the subjects passed with excellent grades, he won't loose any school time. Only in English he had some difficultly, but has promised he will improve. Our little guy is going through all the changes well; I'm proud of him. The transplant hasn't affected him. A girl from the neighborhood is now his best friend. They are both in the same grade and go to the same school.

In a not too pleasant note now, I'm sorry to be the one that has to give you a bad report again Mom. It's about tia Vicky. Apparently when father called her and gave her the news of our imprisonment, she wasn't just shocked, she was fuming mad. Actually Vicky told Dad, "How could Myriam do something so tarnishing to our family's name." It seems she is not ready to forgive you just yet, because she also said, "I don't think I'll write or speak to her ever again." But assured Dad she would look after Grandma and no, Vicky doesn't know anything about my problem!

Father won't mention this incident to you; he figures you are hurting enough as it is. I decided to tell you because you won't be receiving letters from her for a while and her silence will upset you. I'm sure aunt Vicky's attitude will change. After all, she is your sister; she knows the type of person you are, soon you'll have, her understanding and love back. Always remember that creation is based in one word, love. J. P.

Feb. 28th

Dear Mom,

Hopefully all is well with you, as it is with me, but I'm very disappointed in our lawyer. All last week I expected to see Maître Portiere. Unfortunately, he didn't come; he rarely does, though I'm also his client. It must be that I am not that important in the case, which in a sense is good. Still, it shouldn't prevent him from visiting me once in a while, at least to say hello. Ha, ha. Especially since I want to find out what he exactly foresees for you.

It's a common knowledge around here that some lawyers tend to exaggerate the degree of a crime to justify their intended fee; others are more honest. To give you an idea, I'll repeat what I was told about a man caught importing eight kilograms of pure heroin. I'll write the amount in Spanish to make sure you understand, 8 kilos, not 700 grams. He hired a good lawyer for fifteen thousand Francs. At the trial he was sentenced to four years. His lawyer not satisfied with the verdict, appealed. In the appeal, the sentence was lowered to three years. This attorney of course was a true and dedicated lawyer.

The same guys think that in no way your offense could be considered as serious. In their opinion the most the judges will give you, after they'll examine your background is eighteen months. So you see, Mom, you really don't have to worry as much about what Maître Portiere told you. I'm sure these chaps are right. Please keep this in mind and enjoy your weekend.

Love you, J. P.

Life in prison relentlessly continued, even if sometimes I didn't feel much like continuing with anything and my son sensed it. John Paul who was unjustly incarcerated and his own existence hung by a thread because of the disease, yet with an amazing attitude helped me snap out of it with his words of encouragement. In fact, deeply influenced by my son's positive letters and optimism, I ended up thinking alike.

That my offense, was not as serious as what the lawyers implied, in the sentencing aspect that is. All the same, John Paul and I were frustrated; the District Attorney had not summoned us for the interrogation hearing and our attorneys were clueless as to when the inquiry might take place.

At this point, we had two lawyers. My lack of knowledge on judicial matters and the language limitations, seemed to push me from one scrambled situation into another. The reason for the two attorneys was simple, even if the rest was complicated. With the investigation at a stand still, a good lawyer was essential to expedite John Paul's release; evidently *Maitre* Portiere was one. He had the knowledge, consequently was the key person.

Except that in *Maitre* Portiere's next visits, I realized that his English with the heavy French inflection he had, was more than just confusing; actually my comprehension was almost nil. Aware of the deficiency, my husband by means of the Canadian Consul gave me the go ahead to ask Elizabeth to remain on the case. More than anything to serve as interpreter, but also to benefit from the friendship she said had with the District Attorney, which at one point might become handy. Elizabeth accepted but no longer as a public defender; she was to be paid as well, but certainly far less than Portiere.

The tactic seemed good even if came in the form of new impending expenditures. My husband, the same as I, thought that if both attorneys worked together to advance John Paul's freedom and later prepare a good defense plan for me, it would accelerate the results. He just wanted for his son and I to have the best defense that will get us out of France.

While waiting for the outcome and keeping with the *maison*'s routine, something unrelated to the trial came to crank up my spirit. One morning while attending classes, I was called to the workshop. Sylvie, who seemed to be having a major problem with the sewing machine, requested my help. The guard who guided me into the atelier, in need to oversee other duties left me alone with Sylvie.

Yes, at closer range, I could appreciate she was not as young as I thought. Probably in her late thirties, strings of silver had started to show in her blonde curly hair as well as some aging lines at the side of her eyes. A circulating rumor pointed out that she was arrested for heroine trafficking; involved for at least five years. It appeared that a large number of women and men had been implicated in this particular affair, most of them detained now, waiting to be tried. In some of his letters John Paul mentioned it too.

From the few times I spoke with Sylvie, I knew she handled English well. She had a slight French accent that sounded attractive on her, unlike the heavy gibberish Portiere had. As I started to look into the sewing problem, Sylvie spontaneously began to talk about herself and the reason for her detainment. "I'm from Monaco. I'm an only child and my parents are very wealthy. I suppose out of boredom, I started to experiment with drugs from an early age," she said with a childish grin on her face, probably expecting me to say something about it.

Since I didn't, she continued, "I don't know how, or when I became addicted, but soon I found myself using more heroin and cocaine. Later, I even injected myself. At the beginning, the money I got from my parents as an 'allowance,' as you Americans call it, was enough to pay for my needs. As I became more dependent on the drugs, the money wasn't sufficient anymore." Sylvie showed me the scars this addiction had left on both of her arms and continued talking. "I have been an addict for quite some time; did you know?" I shook my head, horrified looking at those hideous marks.

Sylvie, unperturbed, continued with her story. "I resorted to trafficking to support my habit. I got involved with a group of people who carry it out as a business. I was sent to the Middle East and brought the drug back with me. I was paid very well."

Still smiling, she looked at me as if her story was more like a fairy tell than the grisly experience it must have been. Perhaps she just needed to speak giving her point of view, so I quietly listened, "Then Interpol intervened, and over a period of time most of the people involved have been arrested. I'm one, Corinne is another, and many other girls who are here; men too, all jailed for the same offense."

I was not sure why Sylvie would relate such intimate details to a total stranger. Was she trying to attain the same confidentiality from me? Soon I realize, it didn't matter what I said or didn't; she just wanted to share some facts about herself, while I was busy trying to solve the sewing machine's problem.

"In prison, addicts caught trafficking don't get any help from the French healthcare system. As a result I had the most horrible withdrawal symptoms. The moment my parents learned everything, including my imprisonment, they were outraged, but immediately hired an excellent lawyer for my defense."

I wanted to say something intelligent to Sylvie, but I didn't know much about the subject. John and I had experimented with marijuana and cocaine in our social life, so had John Paul, but never had any urge for them, nor considered the harm they could cause. I had seen it happen in movies, but I saw it only as a make-believe situation. This was my first personal contact with someone addicted and I was shocked and silent.

In Bolivia, the production and trafficking of cocaine had increased, but I didn't know anyone who was addicted to the drug. Sylvie's confidentiality opened my eyes to the devastating effects of this dependency. Only because of my imprisonment was I confronted with this reality, which otherwise, I may never have been aware of. Yet in my stubborn mind, I still refused to see myself as trafficker. My motive had been of a totally different nature!

In an hour the guard returned. Pleased to see I had solved the problem she said, "You are handy with sewing machines. Usually someone from the men's side had to be called to make the machine run again. The warden would like to see you now. I'll take you to her office."

The unusual request stressed me. As a rule anything to do with higher hierarchy in this place, inescapably meant trouble. Through conversations with other inmates, I had been clued in that the warden was a tough lady. I had seen her at a distance, but this was going to be my first time facing her and of course I was apprehensive.

I didn't need to be, "Del Castillo, would you be interested in doing some sewing and alterations for the guards in our ward. Or whatever other needlework we might need around here?" she said with what appeared to be a smile. Stupefied I just opened my eyes wide and listened. Her offer came out in fluent English, but she was not done talking. The warden had something else to say, "You will receive a weekly allowance for this work."

I could not believe it. A strange scenario coming from the scarecrow figure the inmates had painted of her. "Sure, I will be glad to do it." Smiling too, I responded immediately. The accord was mutual and the interview ended.

Her request was great. It not only meant I would enjoy the daily showers, but I would also have money to pay a part of the lawyer's fees. In a week or two, after I received my first pay stub, I got another reality check. In prison you are not remunerated the same as in the free world. It showed; I had made just enough to cover only canteen expenditures.

It didn't matter; I had a greater gain. My new position started right after lunch and gave me an unexpected amount of freedom, like roaming around within the two floors of the ward from my cell to the atelier with no questions asked.

Not that liberty was around the corner, no, but following my son's instructions, I found my bearings and mischievously we had unofficial encounters which we called our *prison's escapades*. At the same time John Paul and I tirelessly continued to write to each other on a daily basis, to the wonderment of guards and inmates.

Madame Gonzales became my first customer. She brought the material for a new dress and my success as a fashion designer and seamstress began with her. Soon the word spread and I got more customers, including the Warden. My clientele chose the model from a magazine and without a pattern I converted the picture into the desired dress, attire, or what ever it may be. The guards impressed, treated me with consideration.

In the mornings I kept occupied with the classes, which also helped to keep my sanity intact and my friendship with Claudette grew. Had I not had the judicial part hanging over me, I can honestly say that if John Paul chose to take the incarceration experience as being in a monastery, likewise I felt more like being in a convent. Except for being jammed in the sardine kind of cell, all the rest was pretty much the same as what I knew nuns experienced in their clusters.

With down in the dumps days also came significant up ones, which came in the later part of February bringing a bundle of letters from Bolivia; dated as far back as the middle of January. Likely scrutinized by the D.A.'s dissecting group for almost two months, the reason why it took so long to get into my hands.

One was from my Mom; Vicky was still with her, helping her to cope with the situation and the gossip. Mother, my sweet Mom had the firm belief that I would soon be freed and back in Cochabamba, close to her again. Mother's belief strengthened mine.

Two were from Rose. Mauricio, who had read the Santa Cruz newspaper, told her about my incarceration. She was devastated, but had the presence of mind to let me know the uncomfortable situation Mauricio was going through. Apparently the *voice populi* spread the word saying it was him who had put me up to do what I did; that it was him who was the master mind in the smuggling of drugs. Of course the rumor was false, and he had all the right to be very angry.

Then there were the letters from Mauricio himself who after he learned of our predicament had contacted John, got my prison's address, and wrote to me. His letters brought not only words of concern, but were also filled with anger. He certainly had all the right to be enraged, save for in his most recent one, Mauricio accused my son of being the cause of the problem. In his view John Paul had been the instigator and because of the unconditional love I had for my son, I went along; jeopardizing the factory, the construction business, everything!

He couldn't be more wrong, and how dare he accuse my son? His insinuation made me extremely angry too, to the point that I decided not to answer him. I was sad that he was going through inconveniences and heartaches himself, but Mauricio should have left my son out of the problem. I was not going to neither apologize to him nor explain anything now! I knew I was wrong, but at this point I had more pressing matters to take care of than to be nursing his wounds and that was that!

Judith too had her own setbacks. After over a month of staying in France her siblings, disappointed, went back to the States, leaving her still incarcerated; the so-called friend's promises had not materialized.

Judith and I saw each other in classes and during the promenade breaks, at which time my friend never failed to dump on me all the news she received. This morning she seemed particularly excited, wanting quickly to pass the latest report concerning the woman. I really didn't want to know anything about her, or what she said or didn't, because normally it ended up being questionable and very upsetting for me.

Except that Judith went and blabbed it anyway, as if she had swallowed a canary said, "Lydia has contacted my family in the States and has asked Martha to pay for a return trip to America. She has promised to my sister that things will move more diligently after the trip. Martha immediately bought the plane tickets and Lydia is now in the United States."

All was just too disconcerting and if Judith knew extra stuff about the reason for such a trip, she kept it to herself. What the woman would be brewing now, was a mystery for all concern!

Nonetheless, the next time I saw my son I made him aware of what I just learned, and his mistrust for Judith's friend's as well as mine intensified.

Not Judith's, she still believed in her friend promises. Why wouldn't she? Lydia supposedly was working on her behalf and Judith adamant kept repeating, "No, she had nothing to do with your capture, Myriam"

My annoyance certainly grew, and I my urge to get more information about who this person really was, too? But Judith would not tell me anything more, her lack of response made me wonder again about her own loyalty; showing more interest in protecting her friend's identity than finding the actual facts did not say much for our own friendship!

Besides that, other more pressing issues had me at my wits' end. The famous lawyer I hired because of the great reputation he had, seldom came to see me. How could it be possible that *Maitre* Portiere would conduct himself the same as our legal aid attorney did, not showing up! His indifference or lack of diligence was more than frustrating; what's more, because of the infrequency of his visits, I had not even been able to clarify the topic of his fees.

Elizabeth who was out of sight too made me question about the commitment that both lawyers had for our case. I considered myself intelligent, but probably I appeared dense because of the stupid language barrier, most mortifying to my intellect. Forced to cover all angles, I went as far as to request the Warden to allow Sylvie to act as my interpreter in Portiere's next visit. With her help I had in mind to have a significant conversation with the attorney and spell out all my concerns. Remarkably the warden accepted!

But when the moment came, things didn't start well. As Sylvie and I marched into the room, Portiere who was already there, after his "*Bonjour madame*," totally ignored my presence. The lawyer had come to see me, yet began to talk to Sylvie, about her case instead! Only now I learned that *Maitre* Portiere was the renowned lawyer Sylvie's parents had retained for her, and like an idiot I waited until they were finished their own agenda.

I no longer felt comfortable with the arrangement, but even as infuriated as I was, unfortunately I still needed assistance. As soon as their meeting seemed to be over, I asked Sylvie, "Will you tell *Maitre* Portiere, that before I go any further with his counsel, I need to clarify that I'm not in a position to pay the forty five thousand Francs he requested for his services."

Sylvie, instead of transmitting my concern to the lawyer, volunteered unsolicited advice, "*Maitre* Portiere is an excellent lawyer, Myriam. His defense will be worth more than what he has asked," she openly told me.

All I wanted was to have a straightforward understanding with the lawyer about his fees and my son's release; and lastly about the not showing up issue. I was not interested in her opinion. So politely, but decisively I told her, "Sylvie, will you just translate my words to *Maitre* Portiere, without further comments? I would appreciate it."

She nodded, and after exchanging a few words in French with the lawyer told me, "He has lowered the figure to thirty thousand Francs." I noticed *Maitre* Portiere had said something else in French, but it was left out of Sylvie's translation. Anyway, his response satisfied me.

As soon as this matter was closed, he tried to pull his fast and usual routine; he quickly closed his briefcase and was ready to leave, not discussing anything any further. Up until now without a battle I'd accepted his view on my likely long sentence, but definitely I was not going to sit passively when there were no signs of the positive results he had promised for my son's discharge.

Before he was out the door, controlling my anger, I asked Sylvie to translate, "What exactly are you doing to obtain my son's release?" He uttered some French words then not waiting for Sylvie to interpreter them, in his gibberish English told me "I've been working on it, but you will both first need to be interrogated by the District Attorney. I believe John Paul will be freed at that point." He then waved goodbye and left.

I'd obtained absolutely nothing about dates, or when he planed to come back with more concrete specifics. It was always the same profile; no interaction about our case, no explanations, unnerving to the limit. Could it be that attorneys in France handled their clients in such a distant attitude? It didn't seem possible; at least Judith never mentioned a similar approach in regards to her attorney's performance.

It was more than frustrating; I was tired of a language I could not understand and of lawyers who didn't show one iota of interest in their clients' concerns. Could it be that ours were racists? I supposed I could have just fired them, but there again, I could not afford such bravado. Who would take on our case? Both lawyers were hired to help us, but neither one seemed to be doing anything.

Neither John Paul nor I had knowledge of the French laws or their judicial system, therefore we didn't know what to demand or expect from our attorneys. It was of the outmost importance that my son's innocence be affirmed; sadly, I was not even sure if this famous lawyer believed my words.

Perhaps both legal representatives were only interested in the money, or maybe for them we were just a set of common foreign traffickers who deserved a severe punishment. Who knows? Even if so, weren't they obligated to do something for their clients who had retained them? In my understanding it was in their mandate. In the weeks to come, my frustration and queries grew. The two lawyers I hired to help us, who theoretically were to work jointly on our behalf, simply didn't. Originally they agreed to come together to prepare the case, so that at least Elizabeth would act as the interpreter.

There were no signs of such a team effort. Each one seemed to purposely ignore their commitment. In fact when they decided to show up, each came separately. Their inability to fit their time with each other's schedules was mind-boggling. Elizabeth excused herself from the problem saying, "I have called *Maitre* Portiere several times trying to fix an opportune time for him. He was not available, his secretary took the messages." Supposedly the messages were never answered. Unable to do any more, she left the situation entirely in my hands, as if I could do anything from inside the prison.

As far as *Maitre* Portiere was concerned, Elizabeth was not even trying to coordinate her time with his. Incredible how easy these two professionals could pass the buck to one another, without any consideration for us. When he decided to show up and I asked about my son's discharge, his fixed repertoire was, "I wouldn't worry too much about this Madame Arthur; John Paul will be released at the hearing or right after."

He always knew how to pacify my fury, but time kept going by and nothing positive happened. In other opportunities, the only statement Portiere made sure I understood, was that I risked a long-term sentence, or that the sentences given at The Court of Grasse were harder than in any other district in France. Neither one ever indicated that our case was complex or that John Paul's release could be questioned.

So after a while John Paul and I stop questioning the lawyers' behavior. Maybe we were making a mountain out of a molehill. After all I was the offender, and John Paul was not. Their attitude could only mean that our case bore no complications, which inmates at the male section repeatedly had told my son. Likely they knew what they were talking about!

On the other hand things seemed not to be working out for Judith either. Weeks had gone by and Lydia's promises didn't amount to anything; Judith hadn't regained her freedom. I felt sad for her and I began to warm up to her too. We saw and talked to each other almost every day, in class or at the promenade. She also opened up more and shared her concerns about her children, who were in the States, staying with her sister Martha; and about her husband who was back in Africa and seldom wrote to her.

Then came the day when Inge was liberated and Judith was placed in my cell. We then had the opportunity to have more intimate conversations. I stopped blaming her for my capture, instead setting my pride aside, I asked Judith to forgive me for getting her involved. I believe it was at this point that we became the closest of friends.

During this time together, Judith more explicitly told me about the conversations she and Lydia had, when her friend came to visit her. The woman first had paved the way for her deceitfulness telling Judith, "I'm here to help you. I've a good friendship with the District Attorney and I found a way to arrange your release." Deeply grateful, Judith only saw the kindness of her friend, not noticing the trickery of her next statement, nor in the questions that followed.

"To be able to help you quickly, I need something specific in your favor to bargain with. You probably know more about Myriam's friends, a name or two; or any other people connected with her trafficking?" Those words could not be more conclusive to what she had in mind, but the joke bounced back on her. Judith didn't have any other information to give, because there was none to give. I had no hidden agenda or outlaw skeletons in my closet.

Judith even mentioned that while the woman was in the States, Lydia had the nerve to ask her family to pay for another trip, this time to Bolivia. I presumed she was trying to dig non-existing dirt about me, or if necessary create some; who knows with what in mind? But this time her request was not fulfilled; likely because Judith's siblings realized by now that she was only taking advantage of them and enough was enough.

These details I later shared with my son and soon we had a good picture; the woman's duplicity could not be any clearer. It was then easy for John Paul and I to piece the missing elements of the puzzle together, and impossible not to see the part this woman had played in the affair. We figured she must have set me up from the beginning; too many things pointed in that direction! We were no experts in this field, so we first examined the odds.

288 | Myriam Arthur

She certainly was not an undercover police investigator. A cop would have never requested money from the offender's family for nothing less than to obtain Judith's release, nor to further investigate the case, unless it was a crooked cop which was possible but unlikely. Lydia must have also had connections with police investigators, like the ones that rallied Judith up and have some kind of a relationship with the District Attorney. He was the one who granted the permission to visit Judith in prison

That woman then had to be none other than what in the underworld is referred to as a paid informer. An informer that was not only being paid by law enforcement policing, or whatever they do in France for an exchange of information, but she also obtained fringe benefits by exploiting Judith's distressed family.

Once we had all the clues bundled up, I laid it all out in front of Judith. "You are still imprisoned and your friend has not come back to see you. Added to the other facts you mentioned, it completes the scenario; your so called friend betrayed you, she set the whole thing up from the start." It was only now that Judith finally opened her eyes to Lydia's treachery and saw the full betrayal of her friend. I truly felt sorry for Judith.

In spite of everything an intriguing part of the puzzle was missing, what kind of a tale had this woman fabricated in order to receive the payout, and more importantly for the District Attorney to listen to her story? It had to be something very compelling and detrimental to us. Coming across these particulars did not solve anything, but made us realize that we might be in a battle of preconceived ideas.

Amid this lunacy, what kept John Paul and I still afloat was my husband's comforting letters, a vital source of support. At first John had wanted to come to France and verify with his own eyes that we were well. In addition because he thought his presence in France could help speed up our son's release, except that everything was in limbo; we did not even have dates for the D.A.'s investigation queries, let alone for the trial.

Nothing would have been more pleasing for John Paul and I than to have John's visit. Yet some letters later, we agreed it would only add an unnecessary strain to our already frail finances. Even if the trip was not that costly, and once in Nice John would be permitted to see us often, surely my husband would not be able to remain in France for an undetermined time frame. He had other pressing matters to attend, such as going back to Bolivia to liquidate our assets and the brief happy moments of his visits would instantly pass, making the subsequent separation even more painful.

Just to know that my husband still cared for me, even if he was thousands of miles away, meant a lot, but my mayor as well as instant source of energy renewal were my visits to my son and his letters. But then again, knowing that without a treatment John Paul's life could be soon extinguished, was a torment that never abandoned me. I turned to prayers, but it didn't stop the resentment I began to feel for our lawyers, who uncaringly ignored us.

Assuming that there was nothing complicated about our case, they were still hired to give us legal counsel, even if it only came in an encouragement form. In the middle of all this disorder, we were notified that our first appearance before the District Attorney was set for March 5th. Our attempts to get our attorneys' attention remained the same.

March 1st 1986

Dear Mom, You'll have to excuse me, but this letter is going to be a bit short. I don't feel that good today. I'm run down, tired and even feverish. Even so I still want to send you a few lines and tell you something I have been forgetting to mention before. Congratulation for your new job; I'm happy to know that you are doing the creative stuff you like. Perhaps time will pass more quickly now that you are occupied. I only hope for your sake that the guards are not too fat and ugly, ha, ha

Things do change for the better when people appreciate what we can do for them. Isn't it so Mom? Thank God for the talents we have especially if others can benefit from them. However, you have to be careful. I don't want you to become so indispensable that they might decide to keep you here forever. Oops, I was only kidding Mom. Ha, ha. Seriously though, I'm sure you can easily compete with the creativity of Cartier or Paco Rabane.

Our famous lawyer hasn't come to see me, not even after I sent a strong letter asking him, to explain his view on the case about you and confrontation day is on top of us. Does neither one of them have any respect for us? We are their clients, right? I really don't understand their behavior. However, since we can't do anything about it but wait patiently, and you know this is not one of my fortes, I'm biting my fingernails.

Sorry Mom. I didn't mean to be such a complainer; it must be that I don't feel that good. I'll say by now. I'm going to drink some hot lemonade and go to bed right away. By tomorrow, I'll be okay. Love you, J. P.

March 3rd

Dear Mother,

I have felt so awful for the past two days that I wasn't able to write to you yesterday, not even a few lines. Today I feel better. If you receive this letter before we go to cross-examination, I want you to think positive, be sure that le juge d'Instruction will understand the circumstances of your mistake and by the grace of God, who sees and knows everything, all will go well. Just keep your faith in Him.

This morning I went to Mass, and received the Holy Communion. Afterwards I had a beautiful chat with Fray Regis and I feel ready for whatever happens tomorrow, as I'm sure you do too. We need to be strong. We are God's children and in a moment such as this, He will not abandon us. His presence will be stronger as well as His blessings. You'll see, but you also have to remember that at one time I was told that it could take many months after the cross-examination is over, before the actual trial will take place.

It's during this time, where patience will come in handy; do you see who is talking about it? Me of all people though truly I do feel completely calm and able to face what ever is ahead. There might be a difficult trial in front of us, but we must keep *in mind that no one has ever promised us a bed of roses. At the end we'll find the light but only if we don't lose faith in our Creator. I'll be with you and Judith all the way through. I guarantee we'll all be strong.*

I wish you a very peaceful night, full of God's love. God bless you Mom, your son, J. P.

Through out all this time, John Paul could not have taken his imprisonment more serenely, yet now I was in awe about my son's outlook, even more about the faith and trust he placed in the Lord. Lead by the example of such an inspiring attitude, I was able to control my fear on the outcome of the inquiry and just put the whole lot on the hands of our Lord.

Together with my son's letter, something else came as a surprising and uplifting experience; I received a letter from my sister. Her words were harsh but also forgiving and because it came the day before the hearing gave me another positive jolt.

February 14,

Myriam,

After John called to explain what you had done, I had no intentions to ever write or talk to you again. I felt so humiliated. It was impossible for me to understand how in the world, my sister who had so much success in her life, could have resorted to something so despicable as drug trafficking to obtain money.

If our father would be still alive, the pain and shame of your crime would have been enough to kill him over again. However as the days went by, I couldn't stop thinking of you. After all you are my sister and no matter what, I still love you. I'm sure that when you return to us, you'll explain the reason why you went in that direction.

With the Lord's blessings mother is fine, very sad and concerned about you, but health wise she's okay. I'll be staying with her for a while, to comfort her and watch over her. I just wished this would have never happened, but it has. We now have to pray for this to end, so that we can have you and John Paul back with us soon.

Love you, Vicky.

She was so right! Her reaction was fair. Everything my sister thought about me was true, but unfortunately the damage was done. I was thankful she had reconsidered the situation and her words of forgiveness arrived when I needed them most. Her letter meant so much to me.

MARCH 5, 1986

THE DAY OF THE CROSS-EXAMINATION INQUIRY ARRIVED AND thanks to the boost I got from the letters, I was in good spirits. Judith and I, escorted by two female guards, reached the main gate. Four policemen and two women in uniforms waited next to a van to transport us to the Court of Grasse for the hearing; where we would be face to face with the *le juge d' instruction.*

Inside the van, I saw John Paul handcuffed. Right away the sight deflated my high spirits. Oh how I hated those manacles and there was nothing I could do about them. I gritted my teeth, while with a kiss greeted my son and sat next to him. The officers neither opposed my action nor my choice.

It was an ordinary vehicle and this time there were no escorting cars, or sirens squealing as we drove away from the prison. It felt a bit odd. John Paul and I didn't dare talk; we still had the bad taste in our mouth from the other appalling transfer experience. So it came as a surprise when the sentinels started an amicable conversation that seemed to include us. Just a chitchat talk about the magnificent view in front of us, as the vehicle crossed the city on the way to grasse.

Neither John Paul nor I needed to discuss anything more about the case before the cross-examination. The fragmented input from our lawyers as well as from JP's cellmates, gave us a clear scope about our situation, as a result feeling closer to a happy ending, we just enjoyed the ride! Free from any reservations concerning my son's release, I still intended to add those statements in Judith's favor. I created the problem; it was now up to me to amend it. I had not mentioned anything about it to John Paul; somehow I knew he would rigidly be opposed to the idea.

The beautiful ride ended. We were now at the Court of Grasse and after a short wait we were conducted into the District Attorney's office. Where the men seated behind a desk in perfect Spanish said, "*Mi nombre es Benoit Clavier, soy le juge d' instruction¡ᵃla persona encargada de vuestro caso.*"

My knowledge of court cases was nothing more than imaginary, mainly from watching Perry Mason. So when Mr. Clavier said he was *le juge d'instruction*, which I now understood was the same as a District Attorney, it brought back to my mind that in the T.V. series, the D.A. was the bad guy. The one that always gave a hard time to the interrogated person, individual who in the fiction was actually innocent, but because of the trickery used by the DA, was portrayed as a hard criminal. Until Perry Mason, the attorney for the defense, the good guy showed up and cleared the person.

Elizabeth had mentioned that Mr. Clavier was an understanding person, consequently now his role became conflictive. I didn't know what to expect from him. Mr. Clavier could prove Elizabeth right, or on the contrary could he be the antithesis of her expectations and be like District Attorney in the movies? I would soon find out.

His introduction was followed by another statement: "This cross examination will be conducted in French, translated into English by an official interpreter, for the benefit of the accused, Madame Arthur and her son, John Paul."

Already in knots about the hearing, learning that the interview would be carried out in the two languages I was not savvy in didn't give me any comfort. Then again, I was never asked my preference in the language the questioning should be performed and I didn't have the backbone to lay down the problem, so the audience began.

Something was read in French and after a pause translated to English, "We are now proceeding in conformity with the law and in the presence of the guilty parties opening a sample portion of four grams of cocaine, obtained from the seven hundred grams seized from the personal effects of Del Castillo Myriam and her son Arthur John Paul, by Customs in Perpignan."

The French immersion in which I lived for the past sixty-five days had allowed me to presume that I might have certain understanding of the language, but I did not! Instead that bit of knowledge hindered my awareness, to when it was repeated in English, which was not my forté either, the interpreter's tongue-tied words confused me even more. To complicate matters the strong heartbeat of my heart seemed to obstruct not only my hearing but also my intellect.

Even so I tried to understand, since the audience continued with what appeared to be Judith's first statement given to the police. "We are here now expressly stating the first declaration made before the police in Cannes by the guilty party Judith Del Rey on December 31st."

"When you made these declarations you officially declared and implicated your cousin Arthur, John Paul as the instigator of the importation. There was also the question of you receiving a commission; you acted then in full knowledge of the cause. How do you explain these declarations which in the verbal process appeared to be spontaneously made?"

Not sure if I had heard right, I looked to my son. His pale face confirmed that I heard correctly. John Paul had not only been incriminated in the affair by Judith's testimony, but he actually was pointed as the instigator.

I was shocked! Judith had never mentioned anything about it and from our two lawyers expressions, I could only see their eyebrows raised, sign that they were also unaware of the existence of such a statement, beyond my comprehension.

Instantly I felt no compassion left for my friend and decided that as soon as I had the opportunity, I would tell the whole truth. She was not getting any help from me at this point, but I was not given that chance, because of Judith's response.

She stated: "When I was arrested, I was in a state of shock. Besides that I had promised my *cousine* never to reveal her explanation for the trafficking, namely her son's illness. Back in Bolivia, she had asked me to bring a parcel to France. She didn't specified what it was. Several days later in La Paz, where I went to visit my sick father, I received the tapestries that I ordered in Cochabamba, wrapped and shipped to me by Myriam.

"Unopened I brought the package to France as additional baggage and declared the crafts with Customs. In opening the tapestries at my place, I noticed the extra stuff wrapped inside. It was later when Myriam called me that I was told everything and that the two plastic bottles contained 700grms of cocaine. She then asked me to help her find a buyer.

"My *cousine* told me, she would give me a gift for the favor. It was the police who changed the word gift to commission. They systematically distorted my words. In my first statement to the police, the officers kept changing the gender of the cousin I was talking about. It seems, they assumed and recorded it was my cousin John Paul who initially approached me; when all along I referred to my *cousine*, Myriam, as the one who contacted me."

"Actually when I was questioned, I spoke about both being lodged at my house, but when questioned about the cocaine, all the time I referred to my *cousine*, (female) not cousin, (male). *Cousin* and *cousine* sounds similar; an inaccuracy indubitably made by the police, because of my American accent."

Seemingly Judith used the endearment term cousin, we used as children, even though we were not related. Apparently it was what now created the confusion! On the other illustrated points, Judith had launched herself directly to the part I suggested, to mitigate her offense, improvising a lot and not making much sense.

Yet, when she came to the point to clarify my son's involvement, her response in English, had spelled out the mistake made by the police regarding John Paul's participation. That explanation satisfied me, but her answer led to an unexpected line of questioning.

Q:"Is a true then that you placed the cocaine in your cousin's luggage without her knowledge?" The District Attorney harshly asked me.

A: "Yes." I wanted to tell the whole truth now, but I was not given the chance. Immediately I was bombarded with other damaging questions.

Q: "Do you not have any scruples to have compromised your cousin in such a way that in fact could have significant consequences for her?"

The fabrication was working against me, perhaps even against my son, but I couldn't stop it. I had to back up her story. It would make the case look even worse, if I now declared that all was a lie prepared in her favor.

A: "I do feel guilty, but at that time I didn't think of the consequences. I was desperate because of my son's illness; my only thought was to obtain the means to help him. What's more, if she were caught, I had every intention to assume full responsibility, as I'm assuming right now."

Q: "Why did you put only half of the cocaine in the package?"

The question sounded so out of place. What did it have to do with the other one, anyway? I didn't expect it and I could not just bluntly explain the true facts; that I brought the second part, because I thought Judith had lost the cocaine, she herself brought to France consequent of a trickery. Franticly I searched for an answer that to some extent would make sense.

A: "At the time of her departure only that quantity was ready."

Q: "Who told you your son suffered from AIDS?" The D.A. seemed to be playing a game with me. Now he had jumped into something else, entirely changing the subject again.

A: "It was my son who told me. Our family doctor, who saw John Paul, confirmed it because of the symptoms he presented. But my country lacked the facilities for the specific test on Aids and the doctor is the one who suggested I should take John Paul to France. In his knowledge this country was more advanced in the research of AIDS. What is more, here the illness didn't carry the stigma as strongly as it did in Bolivia."

Q: "The trips you and your son made between South America, the States, Canada and Europe, even the money you invested to purchase the drug, gave us reason to think that the trafficking couldn't be the only financial way to provide the means for your son's medical attention?"

A: "It is true we have holdings in Bolivia. At one point we had the money for those trips, but when I learned my son was ill, my country's economy had collapsed. Money was scarce. It became very difficult to sell anything, if not impossible. Medical expenses abroad are expensive. I was desperate and saw the cocaine as my only alternative. I would have done anything to help my son, so I borrowed the money to purchase it."

Q: "What contacts did you make in order to have your son hospitalized in France?

A: "I didn't make any contacts in France, yet. I didn't know anyone. However, a friend in Spain, a doctor, offered to give us a letter of reference for a colleague in Paris. I needed his advice and the letter to aid us in our search, but I didn't have the chance to pick it up. You can verify the veracity of my claim by calling the doctor."

Without another word, the District Attorney changed course and directed his questioning to John Paul.

Q: "To the accused Arthur, John Paul. Have you been examined by the doctor at the *Maison d'Arret,* and if you have, what was his diagnosis?"

A: "As a matter of fact, yes I have. The doctor said it was possible I had the virus, but no specific tests have been done."

Q: "Why did you tell the police in Perpignan, you thought you were going to Spain to change money for gold, or cocaine?"

A: "I believe the translator misinterpreted my answer. When I was asked if I knew why we were going to Spain, we had just been arrested. Though I knew nothing, by then I had guessed my mother must have done something wrong, which she confirmed only on the spot. Still unaware what it was when questioned, I responded, "she is going to Spain, probably to change something or get some money, but I just don't know what." The word or, sounds like l'or in French, which means gold. Could this be perhaps the reason for the mistake? I never used the word cocaine."

Q: "To the accused Del Castillo, Myriam. Is this true?"

A: "It is correct. Only at the moment of the arrest I told my son I was in trouble."

From somewhere I heard *Maitre* Portiere speak, "The accused Del Castillo, Myriam, wanted to find the cure for her son John Paul, in France, because in Bolivia, France has the reputation of being the leader of research on AIDS."

Finally our famous lawyer had decided to intervene, while Elizabeth kept quiet. After such an incredible input from our attorney the hearing continued without another word from him, or her.

Q: "Now for verification purposes we are showing to the accused Del Rey, Judith and the council, the two manuscript pages spontaneously given to the police by the impeached, and to be noted that the first page is missing."

A:"Yes, those are the two pages I handed over to the police. I don't know what I did with the first page, and don't remember the content."

Q: To the accused Del Castillo, Myriam: Was it you, who wrote the letter? What was in the first page?"

After looking at the pages, I saw it was part of the letter I wrote to Judith from Bolivia with my business proposition, which she was supposedly to have destroyed!

A: Yes. I wrote it. I believe the first page contained only family matters, I don't remember all the details, but in the next pages I mentioned the cocaine."

Q: "To the accused Del Rey, Judith: At the beginning of this interrogation, you answered our questions about your cousin Arthur, John Paul, but in your first interrogation you clearly said it was him who had talked to you about the affair and proposed you to bring cocaine to France. Do you maintain now that Arthur, John Paul was not aware?"

A: "Yes. It was my *cousine* Myriam who talked to me about the service she expected from me. My cousin John Paul never talked about it. I don't know if he was aware of it or not."

Maitre Portiere spoke again: "I would like you to order medical tests to verify if my client suffers from AIDS or not."

The cross examination ended after the counselor's words. I had been bashed from left to right with contentious issues and my dense lies for an excuse probably had further complicated matters. Almost everything was news to John Paul, and Judith's first statement to the police was news to both of us and even to our lawyers. These people who were hired to defend us, how could they have been so irresponsible that they didn't even bother to search and verify any information about the case?

Even now, they hardly said a word in our defense. Wasn't this morally wrong? I never denied being the architect of the whole affair. Unquestionably my offense deserved a penalty, but the allegations presented by the District Attorney, thanks to Judith's first statement to the police, was utterly damaging for John Paul, who was innocent.

On the drive back to the prison, unable to contain my fury I closed my eyes to the guards, to J.P., to everything except her, and I let my pent up anger burst. Had we been alone, I probably would have even jostled her. Somehow I refrained myself and instead I harshly questioned her. "Did the police really make those mistakes Judith, or did you intentionally implicate John Paul?"

She shook her head negatively, tried to say something, but not giving her a chance, I continued. "Why didn't you from the beginning then, stress more strongly that John Paul had nothing to do in the affair that it was only I who proposed the business to you? You know this is the absolute truth Judith, but your explanation didn't sound too convincing to me."

Judith this time quickly interrupted me, "I swear to you Myriam, I told the truth. The police officers were the ones who made the mistake, perhaps because of my American accent, they understood wrongly." She had a good point. Judith's French had an accent, but my anger didn't allow me to listen to reasons. I cut her off again.

"If this is true, why didn't you put more emphasis on exonerating my son, as you did on trying to clear yourself? You even resorted to the story I concocted to make you look less guilty. Now, you better take note Judith, you have the obligation to straighten everything about John Paul, or I'm going to make you sorry for the rest of your life."

Meanwhile, John Paul who had been oblivious to everything unexpectedly spoke, "Mom, it's quite possible Judith is telling the truth. You heard what the police in Perpignan wrote about my answers. They were all twisted around. I'm sure, that even in today's quiz more interpretation blunders were made. What I find unacceptable is the fact that neither one of our lawyers made any effort to clear matters and intervene in our favor."

My son's attitude confirmed what a remarkable young man he was. From day one of our arrest, John Paul who had nothing but shocking experiences, had never uttered a word of complaint. To be implicated now, as the instigator in the trafficking, when he was not even involved, would have outraged anyone else, but not him. Instead, he sided with the person who mistakenly or not, had pointed the accusing finger towards him.

Then to hear Judith's respond at the inquire in a manner that reflected nothing but malice from my part in the affair, corroborated by my own response, was enough to make anyone insane, and John Paul remained unperturbed. Plus to add fuel to the fire he had now witnessed my present quarrel with Judith. Indeed, my son's logic served to cool down my choleric eruption; enraged, the dynamite within me had exploded like a time bomb. I now felt embarrassed.

Obviously the cross-examination continued, each one of us was called to the District Attorney' office, separately and on dates few and far between. My memory and my son's daily letters are the only source to substantiate these hearings; given that all our requests to our lawyers to present us with copies of these testimonies failed; which were extremely critical for verifying the accuracy of the transcripts.

Even at the first quiz, we had established the harmful misinterpretations and blunders made in Judith and JP's first testimonies.

In the later part of March, I was called to the District Attorney's office to a session solely meant for me. *Maitre* Portiere was there. I saw him, but not once did he open his mouth to help. Elizabeth, who had the English background, who allegedly was pals with the D.A. didn't even show up.

Q: "Have you been imprisoned before?"

A: "No. Never in my life."

Q: "According to your own declarations, you do have friends who were imprisoned. Is it because your life is not as honest as you want us to believe?"

A: "I have nothing to hide. As you have said, it's only through my own statement to the police in Perpignan you learned about it. Yes, my husband and I visited two American detainees as volunteers. They did not have any family and had language problems. We felt sorry for them. We provided moral support and some food. That is how I got to know someone who had been in prison."

Q: "I have here two sets of passports, a Canadian one, bearing the name of Myriam Arthur, and a Bolivian one, with the name of Myriam Del Castillo de Arthur; certainly both false?"

A: No, they are not. They are legal documents. I was born in Bolivia. My name is Myriam; my maiden name is Del Castillo.

My husband is a Canadian; his last name is Arthur. When I married him, I became a Canadian citizen. By Bolivian law, I hold duel citizenship"

Q: "Both passports bear stamps from different countries. Was the trafficking the reason for those trips then?"

A: "No. I don't know the span of life these documents have in France, in Bolivia and Canada, they are issued for five years. If you check the dates, you'll find that those trips happened in that period, and certainly not for trafficking. Throughout those years we had the economical means to travel. Our son, John Paul studied Fine Arts at the University of Southern California in Los Angeles, we regularly visit him. My in-laws resided in Calgary, Alberta, Canada; we went to see them, but not as often. My sister and her family live in Peru; we spent sometime with them as well.

The travels to those countries were on family matters. The trips to Argentina and Brazil were on business matters, to buy spare parts for the machinery in the marble factory we owned.

As a person departs the country, it's mandatory for a Bolivian citizen to use the Bolivian passport for taxation and political purposes. I always carry my Canadian one as well. Especially in countries where a tourist visa is required for Bolivians, but Canadians are not, and also because my husband wanted it that way, to avoid political situations."

Q: "Interpol is aware of your trafficking to France. They are now checking your police records in those other countries. What do you have to say about it?"

A: "I'm glad. I wish they would hurry up. It will prove I don't have any offenses in any other country, not even traffic offenses."

Q: "How about the contacts you have in Spain, and also here in France?"

A: "I don't have any other contacts, except the one in Spain. As I told you before, the only reason I resorted to the present trafficking was because of my son's ailment."

Q: "Don't you know you are risking a sentence of at least fifteen years? Why don't you tell the truth instead?"

A: "I'm telling the truth."

Q: "Who packaged the cocaine?"

A: "I did."

Q: "It doesn't seem possible. It was professionally done. Unless you have more experience in trafficking than what you are trying to make us believe."

A: "No one directed or advised me. The idea was my own. I now regret my creativity."

Q: "Stop covering up. We know it wasn't you who master-minded the trafficking; this is the work of a big ring of traffickers! Your son is in on it as well. You both have made this story up. Don't you realize the nature of the sentence you are facing?"

His words hit me as if a hammer had struck my skull. It was not true! I did not belonged to any big ring of traffickers. Why did he insist it was not me who had planned the entire plot? Why did the D.A think I was covering up for my son? Why, did he not accept John Paul's illness? It seemed as though he thought that John Paul's previous trip to France was drug related, not in a search for help and information.

For the life of me I could not figure out any of it. Did he perhaps know something I was not aware off? Could our supposi-tions about the part Judith's friend took in our arrest, not only have been accurate but more damaging than we ever imagined. Why is this man otherwise saying such senseless things? It was obvious his aim was to include my son in my crime, also to make it appear bigger than what it really was, but why?

Could his accusations against John Paul as the instigator, still be based on the misinterpretations in my cousin's first testimony to the police? But, had not Judith said enough to clear my son? Besides he had all the facts that proved the contrary. The cocaine was found in my suitcase, not in John Paul's; the Customs Agents in Perpignan recorded every thing. Then the incriminatory letter my cousin kept, now in the District Attorney's hands, was also part of the evidence. It clearly proved that I wrote it, not my son and Judith had testified to that effect.

306 | Myriam Arthur

From the start, I admitted my guilt. It was not that I was now claiming innocence. It was beyond me, what else did this man want from me? This man whom Elizabeth said had some understanding, but didn't. Whom I had now begun to hate and where was she now? Portiere might as well have not bothered to be present, since there was no input from him.

A: "I have told you everything. I'm telling the truth when I admit I'm the guilty one, also when I say that my son is ill. John Paul plain and simple didn't know anything about my trafficking. I don't care if you sentence me to life in prison; it won't change my guilty plea. What else do you want from me?" I replied, unable to contain my tears.

I could have prevented a lot of pain and anxiety, if from the moment of my arrest I would have just surrendered the truth without any subterfuges. The idiocy of it all was that I had tried to make the investigators understand my circumstances, for breaking the law, without the complete package of the truth and once the curtain had been raised the District Attorney not only acted as the interlocutor, but also as the sentencing judge. This person, who supposedly was the only one in the Court of Grasse who had some understanding, was showing he had none whatsoever.

I wasn't sure if the session had ended because I was crying intensely, or because he didn't have any more questions, but it ended. Immediately after I was driven back to the prison.

On the way back I could not stop crying. My eyes and nose were congested, the thud of the blood rushing through my brain brought about an excruciating headache. I was perhaps on the verge of having a breakdown. Once at the *maison*, when the two guards in charge saw my condition, sympathetically gave me a couple of tranquilizers before I proceeded to my cell. My roommates did the rest, they helped me get into bed, and thanks to the medication a few minutes later I was fast asleep.

I knew from John Paul and Judith that Mr. Clavier was also harsh with them, but never to the extent that he was with me. That man had me terrorized. I had become so afraid of him, that if it was up to me, I would have refused to go to any subsequent sessions, but my son's future or perhaps even his life was at stake, so I forced myself to go.

The sessions were ghastly experiences. In my eyes, the District Attorney was more the executioner than the investigator. He didn't waste a moment in threatening me with a lengthy sentence if I didn't stop covering up. For a while I thought his threats were only directed at me, but because he strongly refused any bail for my son, it seemed he had concluded that John Paul was just as guilty. His tenacity in not wanting to accept the truth of my testimonies was beyond my comprehension. Neither did I comprehend the reasons for *Maitre* Portiere or Elizabeth not doing the job they were paid to perform: to defend us!

I kept asking Elizabeth to bring all the transcribed testimonies to help me understand what was taking place. At a much later date Elizabeth furnished us a copy of the first hearing's transcript. The document enabled us to verify the number of inept translations made at that session; yet it would be the sole record presented to us and only after many demands we made to both of our lawyers.

John Paul and I often wondered, why was she able to obtain that copy, while duplicates of the testimonies we gave at the border but present ones, she was not? Did we have to contend with a specific law in the French judicial system on this subject, or was it just negligence on our lawyers' part? It was a query that remained unanswered.

In one of Elizabeth's visit, I had the opportunity to ask her, "What is really going on? Why is the District Attorney not accepting the veracity of my testimonies and why are you and Maitre Portiere are not helping us in setting the facts right?"

For the first time Elizabeth gave me a short explanation. "Mrs. Arthur, Judith's first statement to the police was very damaging for John Paul; even his own testimony was conflictive. It won't be as easy to clear him now. We will need to prove he is innocent."

"I understand that Judith first statement was damaging for John Paul, but what I don't get it, is why you both were unaware of it; it was important that my son and I knew what we were up against, but neither one of you ever mentioned anything about it. Something else that bothers me is that you know for a fact that a fair amount of what we said in English, once translated and recorded into French had many incorrect interpretations. You are well versed in French and English, why then didn't you correct or at least say something about it for the record?"

"Here in France, lawyers are very limited in the amount of intervention we are allowed to have on behalf of our clients. We are not as privileged as the attorneys in America, where the judicial system permits their input at all times." Elizabeth tone of voice sounded apologetic as she recited her excuse.

We often wondered if this was a true fact, or if it was another one of her fibs to justify their negligence; difficult to verify it since we had no one in France to give us an accurate response on the subject. All we knew was that everything was just out of proportion. To be treated as hard-core criminals, where the head of the gang, me, had no foot to stand on. It was ludicrous.

Some loose ends about Judith's friend's intervention kept coming to my mind. It probably had a lot to do with the D.A.'s attitude. It brought a different perspective on the way things were developing. It was probably me, who early on had given the woman powerful as well as misleading information that only now began to bring some light in my eyes onto the situation.

When still in Bolivia and I had first approached Judith, she had posed some questions which Lydia had wanted a response from me. At the time both her inquiries and my answers seemed harmless, "What quantities is your cousin talking about" she had asked, and without a second thought my response had been, "Seven hundred grams, to start."

As time went by and neither action nor results came, and looking only to my son's condition and my need to bring him to France, I told Judith to threaten Lydia with these words, "You better tell your friend to hurry up, or I will sell the stuff to someone I know in Spain."

Even later on, as we were leaving for France, I harshly rebuked Judith. "You don't have to worry about the powder any longer; the problem won't be yours anymore. I'm going to pick it up and I will take care of the stuff myself. A friend in Spain will purchase it, plus what I'm bringing too." Unquestioningly Judith repeated my command word by word to her friend.

Damaging statements in the wrong hands! Sounded extremely accusing, as if a ring of traffickers were in operation, when it was only the bravado of a desperate mother. They were words spoken out of fear, frustration, and anger that possibly now were coming back at me. All this fitted perfectly well with the rest of the puzzle; she only had to add a few more words of her own invention to have the full attention from the D.A. and by the look of things it appeared she had succeeded.

There was no other explanation for the harshness the District Attorney had with us; still, everything referred to my plot, to my involvement, not to John Paul's. All the more like a daunting movie than a reality.

To pacify myself, I continued with my one sided conversations with The Lord and I did most of the talking. "Father, you see and you know everything, so you are aware that John Paul is innocent. Please, I beg you, use your powerful intervention and open Mr. Clavier's eyes. His dire attitude is unfair, will you please do something about it!"

When things went from bad to worse, I pleaded more vehemently, "Lord, I've acknowledged I offended you; not once, but a thousands times. I also know that after I confessed my sins you forgave me. So, why does the punishment remain? Can't you see that I have had enough?"

As a norm Rev Regis, who came every week, knew of my dialogues with our Father, also the deep hatred I had developed towards the District Attorney. Wanting me to contain it, he suggested I recite with him the one and only prayer taught by Jesus to his Apostles good and helpful at all times.

Our Father who art in Heaven, hallowed be Thy name, thy kingdom come, Thy will be done on earth as it is in heaven, Give us this day our daily bread; Forgive our trespasses as we forgive those who trespass against us, and lead us not into temptation, but delivered us from evil. Was there a response from Interpol? No idea. Our lawyers didn't mention anything; they seemed as clueless as we were about it and on the whole thing for that matter. Maybe that investigation had not even been requested and was just another way for the District Attorney to intimidate us, to waste time. We actually looked forward for the report to be in the District Attorney's hands; it would prove that our lives were flawless before the situation here in France.

Relentlessly time kept going by and by the Lord's grace, John Paul's health was still okay except for some bronchial colds with elevated temperature, but fortunately as fast as the problem started, with the antibiotic treatment he was given, right away the malady abandoned its lodging too. While all this took place not once I hear a word of reproach from John Paul. On the contrary, he always managed to uplift my spirit through the flow of his loving letters and the happy characters he drew.

March 24

Chere Maman,

I hope you feel better now, after all the rubbish the District Attorney dumped on you yesterday. The important part is that you survived, that is what counts. The man is insane; one day he will render account for all the cruelty he is leaving behind. You just wait and see, Mom.

I think it was the influenza what got me down for a bit, but I'm now fine, just overly impatient from the lack of news from Interpol. For a change Elizabeth came to see me today and I had the opportunity to ask her something I had on my mind, "Would it be acceptable to contact people back home, and ask them to write reference letters? From important persons such as Monsignor Morales the auxiliary Bishop in Cochabamba, who knows our entire family's background and can vouch for us. Also other ecclesiastic authorities that have ordered marble for their churches and know my Mom from her work at the factory, and friends, they can give surety on her integrity. About myself, I asked if records from my University and my work would help?"

She approved the idea. Elizabeth thinks documents such as those would be very helpful in the investigation, later even at the trial. You can't image how happy I'll be to see le juge's face, when he finds out the kind of people we truly are. Going a little ahead of myself, I also asked her, if once I was acquitted could I be allowed to remain in France until you have completed your sentence. She didn't see any reason why not.

I am writing to my university, also to Universal Studios asking them to send all my records, grades and job description to the District

Attorney, better yet to Dad. He will make sure the certificates and the rest will get into the proper hands, our lawyers, so that I have something positive in my favor too.

I suggest you have the Canadian Consulate call Dad. It will be faster. He then can contact Grandma and explain our need for the letters, the sooner the better. Mom, believe me the letters will be like a slap in the D.A.'s face. Soon he will have to apologize for his bad behavior with us. Ha-ha.

Now I must say good-bye. I need to hurry up and take care of my letters.

I love you. J. P.

March 25th

Dear Mother,

The letters have departed. Now, to cheer you up I'm enclosing a portrait I drew of Patrick. I had a small picture of him and used it as a model. I thought it would give you a great pleasure to have my brother by your side as well, even if it's only a replica. Ha, ha.

J.Pecito, the small character I created to keep you company in good and sad times, is coming to visit you. This time, besides his big smile he is

*carrying his Viking sword to fight off our enemies,
such as the District Attorney has turned out to
be. You have my promise Mom; you won't have
to be afraid of that man anymore, because your
warrior, J.Pecito, will be on the lookout to protect
you from him, as he is doing in this letter.*

Looking forward to see you soon,

Love, J. P.

Such a brilliant idea; the D.A. would necessary have to accept the facts once the letters were in his hands. If our defense lawyers would have been on the ball, the suggestion should have come from them, but it did not why? My previous concern about them came back. Did these lawyers even believe us? Or for them were we just some low class people, drug traffickers, who therefore didn't deserve their attention?

At least something positive was in the works and Elizabeth was not opposed to my son's strategy. She actually agreed that the investigation would speed up with such documentation. For my part, I followed John Paul's suggestion. I asked Patricia to contact the Canadian Consulate with the following message for John. "Mr. Arthur, your wife and son need to obtain reference letters from Bolivia and California. It would be best if they come, from religious, political and business people in Cochabamba, people that can vouch for Myriam's character. For your son, records from his university and his work the sooner the better. Once you have it all send it to Maitre Portiere."

My husband went into high gear; he immediately contacted the Royal Canadian Mounted Police and requested criminal record checks for both John Paul and I. He also called my mother for all the Bolivian documents and Patty, our son's friend in Los Angeles for Californian papers.

In return mail, John received the police certificates showing that John Paul and I had clear records in Canada. My cousin Raul keenly helped my mother in all the diligences and she attained similar certificates from the Bolivian police force. Ecclesiastics and other important people in the business world, anxious to assist, wrote the requested testimonial letters. The political authorities politely declined; intercede in a drug trafficking related issue was not permitted in their capacity, no matter how well they knew us.

Official interpreters at the Consulates translated the letters and documents into French; all bearing the seal of the offices in Cochabamba and Los Angeles to make the translation official and without delay they were sent to my husband.

Once John had them, he forwarded all the documentation by certified mail to *Maitre* Portiere; enclosing a pleading letter to the District attorney on my behalf, which the lawyer was to deliver personally. My husband had the signed receipt of reception in his hands, dated April 9; therefore the parcel definitely reached the attorney before the investigation was over. His job was to hand everything over to the District Attorney. We presumed the mission was completed. The decent thing for the D. A. to do now was to rectify his mistake and release John Paul.

Nothing happened. We began to wonder if Mr. Monsieur Clavier would ever accept anything other than what he already assumed. A few weeks later, Elizabeth opened my eyes; it was not entirely his fault. "Madame Arthur, Mr. Clavier hasn't received those documents. I've just spoken with him yesterday. I asked him about it, since you mentioned Maitre Portiere should have already presented them over to the D.A." Elizabeth's words came in her exasperating quiet usual way, more unnerving for me now, after what I had just heard.

"What!!! You mean to tell me that Portiere hasn't presented this valuable information? Is he out of his mind? How can he be so negligent! He knows the same as you, the importance of establishing our background's integrity before the District Attorney," I exploded; fire flames shooting up from inside me. It was just too unfair. For the life of me I could not understand under what kind of principles the attorneys worked in France. But according to Elizabeth's next words, there was a perfect explanation,

"Mrs. Arthur you shouldn't be so upset. *Maitre* Portiere is well-known for keeping this type of evidence in favor of his clients as a last minute resource, at which time he feels it has a more favorable effect." Candidly, or stupidly I believed her. We should be able to trust our lawyers after all. Her reassuring words made sense. I discussed the situation with John Paul and even he, thought it was a good move.

In the mean time, Josee, who was still the number one news-wizard at the *Maison,* brought to the cell shocking news. "Two Colombian young women have been arrested at the international airport in Nice, but they are in the hospital now. They seemed to have swallowed small rubber cartridges full of cocaine in Colombia and carried the stuff in their stomachs, very dangerous. If one of the devices bursts they wont be around to tell the story. If they survive, the girls will be placed here!" she coldly explained.

The Colombian cartel's technique was well known in the prison's milieu. Out of necessity people were contracted as mules, a word that described persons who transported the drug in this manner. Drug traffickers often resorted to this terrifying method to obtain fringe benefits from the illegal trade and these young women were put to the task endangering their lives.

A few days later as Josee stated, the Colombian girls made it through the ordeal and were now in *la maison d'arret.* I saw them at the courtyard. They didn't look older than nineteen or twenty and seemed very scared. Fresh in my memory the fright of my own arrival, instinctively I reached out to them trying to ease their situation.

Elena and Fanny opened up too, especially Fanny. Still shaky from the test, she told me what actually happened, "Before we

left Colombia, we swallowed a bunch of small rubber recep-
tacles packed with cocaine. Once in Nice, nature should take its
course and at that point someone would contact us, to reclaim
the product and pay us." Elena remained silent while her friend
talked, but held her hand in support.

Fanny encouraged continued with their story. "It didn't happen
as planned. While going through Customs, our nervousness must
have given us away, because we were commanded to go through
an x-ray machine set at the airport. The capsules were instantly
detected and we were placed under observation and cops watching over us, until we eliminated the pebbles. We are here now and
have no idea what will happen next?" Fanny concluded. I could
not say much to console them, since I didn't know where my case
stood either. I just became a friend.

Something similar happened in Paris a while back; again, it was
Josee who mentioned the incident, but the situation here was different it touched me. I met the girls involved in the offense and
for the second time while at the *Maison*, I was faced with the
brutal reality of the harm drugs and traffickers cause on people,
in the pursuit of the mighty dollar.

I was shocked; perhaps I was no different from those common
traffickers. Had I not resorted to the same, because I needed
money? Early on, I got away from my conscience's reproach, in
the belief that my motive gave me the right to follow the old adage,
"*The End Justifies the Means.*" Obviously, I now had a clearer view
of my offense.

At this point Fray Regis words' made more sense; my Father in
heaven was making a strong point. In my time in prison, I was to
learn the miseries drugs brought to people. Further yet, I needed
to open my eyes to where my own life had been heading. Had I
not been caught, how much damage the cocaine I brought would
have caused? How many lives would have been destroyed, even if
I had saved my son's?

I accepted this lesson, but I also rebelled. John Paul shouldn't
have been brought down along in my misery. The instruction was

loud and clear; consequently the lesson should be over now. It was too unjust for my son to suffer a penalty for his mother's fault!

In any event the arrival of the two girls brought a change. Both attended classes and at the promenade we talked a lot, about their families, while I chatted about John Paul. Fanny got interested in him and the same went the other way around. J.P., also curious about this cute Colombian girl, asked me to tell him more about her.

I suppose the detainment tediousness influenced John Paul and Fanny to try their luck and requested permission to write and visit each other. The corresponding was approved, not so the visits. In any event J.P. and Fanny began exchanging letters and enjoyed every bit. It was a welcome change for both.

Then unavoidable realities brought me in crash landings too. Such as when I learned that John was forced to sell our beautiful unfinished house at below cost. It was to avoid the foreclosure the loan shark had tried to put on the property for lack of payments. Had Victor succeeded, he could have kept the house for next to nothing. My husband's steps stopped it.

John's own dire financial situation also forced the outcome. His parents had lent him the money for the lawyers' retainer fees and they needed it back, credit cards were maxed out; all needed to be repaid. Besides it was costly to carry on life in Canada without a job. Even if John and Patrick were lodged at my husband's parents place for free.

Quesnel was a small town in northern B.C., that had nothing much to offer, not for my husband anyway, who was looking for work. Resumes went and appointments for interviews were made, as a result John repeatedly had to displace himself, to Vancouver in B.C. or Calgary in Alberta, where most mining corporations and oil industry had their head quarters.

None of his efforts paid off; in his years of absence from Canada, John had lost contact with companies and people, the link he needed to succeed in his hunt. From his letters, I sensed the devastation this brought to his pride; for the first time in years, my husband was unable to find work.

Frustrated John went back to Quesnel; my husband didn't feel right to be far from our younger son for too long either. My in-laws were elderly and John had not told them anything. They believed their son and I had some issues that needed time to work it out. It was at this point that John saw no other alternative than to resort to the quick sale of our house in Bolivia, below cost.

My mother, provided with his power of attorney, proceeded with the sale. My husband had more than enough worries on his hands and our situation in France made matters even more difficult on him. Caught in a vicious circle, he was unable to dedicate enough time to find a job, the work he so badly needed!

Naturally the losses and my husband's frustration weighed heavily on me. It was a disastrous shortfall, but the setback was overshadowed by an even greater concern. The District Attorney finally had ordered John Paul to be tested for AIDS, as well as have him go through a thorough medical assessment.

Eleven months had gone by since I first learned John Paul had been infected and my knowledge of the illness was as stagnant as ever. It could not be otherwise being imprisoned. Except that John Paul now often had periods of swollen glands, high body temperature, even some bronchial problems, distinctly symptoms related to AIDS. "Healthy people have them too," I reasoned. Undoubtedly hoping against hope that my son's suspicion of having contracted the virus was just a big mistake.

As the layperson that I was, when the tests returned with the diagnosis that John Paul was HIV positive, the threat that hung over my son's life came back full-blown. I still had no notion of the difference between HIV and AIDS.

At this point I could not just stand idle and let the District Attorney's unfounded suspicions be a menace to my son's health any longer. The man was unshaken and worse yet, our lawyers didn't seem to be doing anything to assist us.

Determined I decided to seek help elsewhere, so I wrote to the European Commission of Human Rights in Strasbourg, soliciting advice and help. Their response didn't take long to arrive. The commission sent me a booklet pertaining to what these human rights were, and when it was possible for the European Commission to intervene. Unfortunately, my demand didn't meet their criteria, and therefore my request for their help ended there.

Someone among the inmates made me aware that Madame Danielle Mitterrand, the wife of the President of France, Monsieur Francois Mitterrand, was a good-hearted person and that I should try appealing to her. This was likely politically incorrect, but at that point, I didn't care. All I wanted was to obtain outside help for my son's situation. With all the respect to her high position I wrote to her. I explained what I had done and the result my action had brought upon my son, begging her, as a mother as she herself was, to intercede on my son's behalf.

Madame Mitterrand's response came in a letter dated July 30, written by her private secretary. She stated that it was impossible for Madame Mitterrand to intervene in justice affairs.

At the same time, I had addressed President Mitterrand himself. Monsieur Mitterrand's response arrived August 25, written by *Le Conseiller Technique*. It stated that my letter had been passed on to the Justice department, but nothing came from that department either.

Then I remembered Regis Debray, now a well-known French politician, who, in 1966 acting as a news reporter was incarcerated in a Bolivian prison. Suspected to be a member of an irregular paramilitary unit, he was taken prisoner jointly with a group of the guerrillas commanded by Che Guevara. After almost two years of incarceration, and thanks to the intervention of the Bolivian Human Rights group and the French authorities, Mr. Debray was released.

Somehow I obtained his address and I wrote to him as well as to a cousin, who was one of the officials of the Bolivian Human Rights group, he had been instrumental to his release. I asked him to write to Mr. Debray on behalf of my son, too. The two letters were sent in the hope that as a person who had passed through the pains of an unjust incarceration would understand our situation and would act accordingly.

I was not asking clemency for me, by now I already knew I would need to pay harshly for my crime. My plea was for my son, who was an innocent party but maybe the address was wrong; or the letters never arrived to his hands. In any event neither my cousin in Bolivia, nor I, ever received a response to our letters.

Everything I tried and hoped it would bring help to clear my son had failed. His unjust incarceration was more painful that what I could bear! I just could not understand how a situation as the one we were going through, could take place in a civilized country like France. I had admitted my guilt several times over, why then the rest?

As I saw all the doors closed, and that all my efforts to clear my son before the trial hadn't amounted to anything, I decided to go on a hunger strike, hoping my protest would be heard. I supposed through Fanny the information must have leaked to my son, and John Paul's immediate reaction came in a concerned letter.

Friday, July 31

Querida Mamita,

You must forget the crazy idea of going on a hunger strike. Your plea won't even be heard, and you'll only end up hurting yourself. The boys here tell me that you must put that idea out of your mind, because, here in France this method doesn't work. The authorities supposedly could care less whether you eat or not; or die for that matter and the damage would be only to your health. Besides,

I believe we should wait and see what comes from the French judicial system and from our lawyers. If injustice prevails, at that time we can always refer to The Human Rights in Strasbourg again.

In the meantime, Mom, don't worry anymore. This doesn't mean that we should allow depression or resignation to overpower us. Recently, I was starting to feel that way myself, seeing me as just another prisoner, which I'm not, and will never be. I'm an unjustly detained person and that is it. At one point I told you, I would gladly take the blame, but that was a totally different story from what is happening now.

I hope you and Judith are able to face this problem, with prayer and positive thinking, with God's help and the love of our family; we will be able to bear anything this unpleasant chapter has brought into our lives. We will all be together again, and more united than ever.

Mi amor por ti mama, es para siempre. J. P.

Whether my son's admonition was correct or not, I accepted it. The next time we were together, he actually told me, "Mom you need to promise me that you will never go on a hunger strike." So I did, but to see my son not freed in the course of the investigation, as the attorneys assured me would happen, left me with an inferno inside me.

All my hope now rested on the trial. On the judges, who with every single fact in their hands should realize that my son had been wrongfully accused! I prayed intensely for God to open their eyes!

In the mean time, not everything at the *maison* was dark or doomed. In fact even though the conditions of the habitat were not the best, but in all honesty I can say that for the most part John Paul and I not only found warmth and understanding among the inmates, but also sensed a favorable attitude from everyone involved in our surveillance. I felt protected in la *maison*; the ghastly cross-examination hearings with the D.A. and his heartlessness could not penetrate the thick prison walls. It was more as if I were in a cloister instead of in a prison!

Our social workers were considerate and helpful. The support and sympathy my son and I found in our French teachers was closer to a friendship. John Paul's professor impressed with his art, went the extra mile to have him paint a fresco in the classroom, also to be the one doing the drawings for the prison's internal journal. He knew how much this signified for J.P.; plus a small economical remuneration and the daily showers. My son, with no thoughts of his own situation found incredible ways to make me feel his closeness.

To keep me amused, under his directorship we played games. We both pretended to be in boarding schools, where the guards played an important part. Supposedly they were severe nuns and monks, but only too anxious to show their good hearts. While in the game, it progressed into some mischief and a few times we got caught in the act. Neither John Paul nor I were ever disciplined for our mischief; likely recognized for what it was, children acting up.

My sewing became a regular job. In the mornings I attended classes, and I worked in the afternoons. I had clients galore; my best ones were the Warden, Madame Gonzales and Véronique, a female guard from John Paul's side, plus sometimes other regular guards. Everyone was satisfied with my work, including myself. I earned a little money, and made them happy. I increased their wardrobes with fancy new outfits or altered old ones into more fashionable ones. The best part for them was that they didn't have to pay me a dime.

My son had compared my abilities to Paco Ravan's. Just for the fun, I decided to make John Paul intangibly participate in some of my clients' try-outs. Play-acting I told him, "Envision the Warden in one of the fitting sessions. Madame the In-Keeper comes and after all the preliminary greetings, I'm the one who tells her, "You need to take off your clothes," mind you, only the uniform and not to perform the well-known search, but to let her try the dress. It was a little bit, like getting even! Ha-ha." J. P. loved when I could joke, and I was not consumed by worries.

Thanks to my sewing talent, I enjoyed a place of privilege. Our model cell was kept unlocked during certain hours of the day. They no longer needed to run back and forth to unlock our cell, to let me out to go to the workroom. It helped that my roommates had a very good reputation as well.

The unlocked door was an unexpected gift. It gave me the freedom to come and go as I pleased. It was not that I could just walk out of the prison, this would have been impossible; ten barred gates were in my way. Besides, even if I could, how could I even think of running away knowing my son was left behind!

But it enabled me to freely walk to the window in the hallway, next to my cell. The one my son so many times had pointed out to me. From where, placing a chair under and standing on it, I was able to slightly see his figure plastered on a small window a short distance away, but able to hear his voice loud and clear. Miraculously, I found my bearings and we had some fun.

John Paul, the minute he started to work had free access to the communal showers. Where using his acrobatic skills would climb onto the high windowsill and patiently wait for me to show up. Of course we had already established a time schedule for these rendezvous. The remarkable window became like a citadel for mischief.

At the set time, on tiptoes I stood on the back of the chair for the adequate height. Then J.P. and I would exchange signs of affection and bits and pieces of conversation, while my roommates remained on the lookout, in case any of the guards unexpectedly showed up at the scene of the crime. It was while doing this choreography that a few times we were caught, but only received gentle reprimands, by this time I believe every one involved in our supervision, inmates included were on our side.

When back home, we used to enjoy every movie Steven Spielberg directed. "Close Encounters of the Third Kind," was one of them; J.P. was so attracted to the work of the director as well as to the industry. So now for fun while in the action, he pretended to be the director of our own movie, which he called "The Secret Encounters of the Prison World." Every day, a few minutes before noon and at four o'clock, a new episode was filmed.

It didn't matter that we saw each other just for a few seconds; what was significant was that these flashes made J. P. and I feel like we still held some control in our lives. Besides it was amusing to act like two mischievous children. We took some risks, true, but for those split seconds we were able to forget the reality of our imprisonment. It reminded me of some of my childhood naughty times at school.

And here we were now, John Paul and I, playing games like a couple of kids, hoping not to get caught, while having a little amusement. J. P. had made many friends with inmates who work in different areas. One of them, worked in maintenance, he had drawn the building plan of our wing and this is how my son became familiar with the layout of our accommodations.

John Paul 's resourcefulness was unlimited, even if his surroundings were not, and found other ways to make me feel his closeness. At times a special messenger sent by J.P. came calling under the small window in our cell; a whistle was the calling card. Forewarned in advance, I was to throw a string through the window and pull it back up once I felt a tug. I always found a flower attached to the other end. The messenger was one of the prison's gardeners, a young African inmate, also good friends with J. P., so I became his Mom too!

Apparently twice a year a group of Christian Rock Band Players came to the *maison* to perform for the inmate population. I understood that they had sung on the males' side a couple of days earlier and on August 12th the band paid a visit to our wing. The musicians played and sang a number of beautiful Christian songs; following their catchy tunes we all chanted with them.

For some reason their repertoire included a Happy Birthday. Through the loud music, I heard repeatedly a name; it sounded like mine. Once the song ended, one of the young men from the group, through the speaker said, "Will Myriam stand up please; we want to say a few words to the person for whom this song was dedicated."

There was no other Myriam than me. So I stood up, a little embarrassed for the attention I was receiving. Then the singer spoke again, "You must be a very special mother. Your son went to a lot of trouble to have this song delivered to you today. In fact, we were supposed to have come here on a later date, but he insisted that it had to be the twelfth of this month. We are very happy to have obliged him. Happy birthday, Myriam! From what we know, your son's effort and ours will bring joy to your heart on this important day. God bless you."

Too overwhelmed by the unexpected surprise, I was unable to even thank them, but I was sure they understood my silence and my tears.

Those were our fun times. Unfortunately John Paul and I still had to face the other side of the French judicial system, and the one outside the prison's walls was not pleasant. The District Attorney had not changed his attitude. He continued to treat us like hard-core criminals. His injustice with regards to my son ignited in my heart a deeper hatred for him which I could not restrain.

"Love thy enemy" was not working for me, not with respect to the D.A. anyway. The investigation ended in the second part of

July. As far as we knew our situation had not changed, not in the eyes of the District Attorney anyway.

In the latter part of August the trial of the large ring of drug traffickers ended. Involved in the circle were over sixty people. Sylvie and Corinne, the two inmates who served the meals were in the midst of them. From this large group only forty were tried. The rest had fled the country. Among those who fled was the leader, tried in absentia and condemned to eighteen years in prison, the second in command to fifteen years.

Others of high rank received between eight to ten years; this was a true ring of drug traffickers. Sylvie was sentenced to six years, Corinne to four, while the rest received minor sentences and some were even acquitted. Through our French classes we had access to the local newspapers and according to the media the trafficking had been going on for over five years, and enormous amount of profit had been made.

Reading about the affair, John Paul, Judith and I could not but compare this crime with our own situation. If habitual offenders after years of trafficking, with profits made from right to left were handed these sentences, we who had no previous offenses would certainly be dealt with in a minor degree. John Paul acquitted, since he had no part in the offense. Judith could not be sentenced to more than a year and I, the head, the leg and the arm of the plot to a maximum of four; even though there was never much of an operation.

August 29th, the three of us were served with some legal papers stating: "The investigation of your case has now been closed. It's been ruled that there is enough evidence of trafficking in French territory for less than three years, especially in Mandelieu-Cannes, on December 31st. You will be tried at a future date at the Court of Grasse."

Finally! The investigation was closed, but still we had not made any headway with the District Attorney. We now only counted on the fairness and understanding of the people who held seats as judges and were so placed to impart justice. Anxiously we waited for that date, which was still a hidden agenda, and the months continued to roll by.

In the months following our arrest, none of my relatives or friends except for my mother and sister, as well as Mauricio and Rose, had written to me. I didn't hold it against them; probably they had no idea how to tackle the problem. Putting myself in their shoes, I would not have known what to say or do either. Anyway it was best that way. There would come the day when I was free, and I would then have the chance to discuss my situation in depth with them and Mauricio especially.

So now eight months after my arrest I was taken aback when I received a letter from my cousin Raul. Before I even opened the letter, my first thought, went to my mother. Was she perhaps ill? He had promised my sister to keep a watchful eye on Mom.

Through out my entire life, Raul had showed only integrity and profound moral values. Except that in earlier years, my sister and I didn't see things eye to eye with him. In our view cousin Raul acted the same as the cloister nuns from our school. Always finding faults in our *charming* dispositions.

"It is not good to be facetious; boys will have a wrong concept of you if you keep this up," he would say. I am sure he meant well, but at the time we didn't appreciate it. Instead we considered Raul too dogmatic, the same as some of the nuns and priests who we found had remained static and outdated, not wanting to go along with the life changes.

The letter had nothing to do with my mother. Raul's missive only indicated, "Lila and I are going to Barcelona to visit our son Santiago. He is studying there for the priesthood. We are going to try and extend our trip to Nice. We want to see you." I was sincerely ashamed of what I had done, but I dreaded the thought of seeing them. I was not ready to accept criticism. Nor tell anyone outside my immediate family the reasons for my behavior, let alone him.

I had not heard from Raul any further. He probably had a busy schedule on his hands. Swinging like a tornado in an out from business appointments, had ran out of time and was unable to come; a great relief for me.

Until one Saturday, around 10 a.m., a guard gave me a jolt, when she came to my cell and said, "Myriam, you need to descend. You have a couple of people waiting for you at the *parloir.*" Those were the booths designated to receive outside visitors.

In fact my cousin and his wife had arrived in Nice on the weekend but were unaware that they needed a special permission to see me came directly to the prison. Amazingly the staff handled the crisis in a most unusual and superb way; they understood the situation and made their visit possible.

I wished I could say I felt confident. But no, as I walked to the tiny reception room, my legs were a bit wobbly; the cause could only be Raul's visit. I didn't know what to expect. A long sermon as the ones he used to give us when my sister and I were young-sters? And to boot I was now in prison!

Before I knew it I was in front of them; my entire defense tactic failed as my cousin embraced me. From his tender expression, I realized Raul had not come to judge my actions. My cousin's detour to Nice was only to give me his love and support. After, his wife Lila also embraced me and my protective barrier came down completely. For the next few minutes we just held hands and shed many tears.

He had no words of reproach, only concern. At one point however my cousin asked me, "Why did you do it Myriam?" Without hesitation, I responded, "I'm sorry Raul; I can't answer your question. Not now, but I promise you, soon you will know the truth." No one except for John and Patrick knew John Paul was sick and I was not about to break the silence just yet.

Back home, Raul who was a very busy entrepreneur had offered my mother his assistance. I knew he had kept his vow. He had even taken time from his businesses to help my mother secure the testimonial letters for our defense. I had a lot to thank my cousin for.

Their visit lasted for a little more than one hour and it became a most rewarding experience. As they were leaving, Raul said, "As soon as I'm back in Cochabamba, I promise to report to your mother. I'll reassure her that you are well and from what you have informed me, John Paul too. I know how concerned *Tia Lia* is. I'll make sure my report eases her mind a little. Unfortunately, I have to hurry and attend business meetings in Paris and Belgium. I will not be able to come back, nor visit J.P.. Would you please give him our love?"

It seems that with the good, something unforeseen always follows. I was still taking pleasure in my cousin's visit, when in the later part of September; through a letter from Patrick, I learned John had been hospitalized. A new growth had developed in his bladder, which the same as in 1982 turned to be cancerous. September 16th the growth was surgically removed and thankfully the prognosis was good.

Once on his way to recovery my husband made sure to send the pertinent medical documentation to *Maitre* Portiere, along with another letter to the District Attorney. Letter in which, John begged him clemency for his wife and justice for his wrongly accused son! Short of any acknowledgment, we assumed the D.A. either ignored the data, or Portiere chose not to present the package. It was impossible to know from behind bars.

The September surprises didn't end there. The 20th, we were notified the date of our trial. It was set for Friday, October 13th, 1986. Neither my son nor I had superstitious tendencies, but Judith became paranoid with the date and challenges did not end there, in fact more were in the works.

The next unforeseen event was destined solely for me. At the very beginning of September, I had detected a painful lump in my left breast. My mind occupied in more important issues, didn't put much attention to the pebble. Still it was something I could not just ignore, so I mentioned it to Madame Gonzales. Advised by her, I signed a request to be seen by the doctor that came regularly to *la maison*. He checked me and the lump was probably of some concern, because he told me a surgery would be schedule for the immediate future.

What a blasted situation! We finally had a set date for our trial and the stupid operation could become an unexpected obstacle. I knew, I would not need to think twice if that were the case, I would forego the surgery. The trial had to be over and done with without any more delays; John Paul had to be set free. If in all this time the District Attorney stood in the way, I was sure the person tasked with judging us would have a more objective mind. They would see the strong evidence validating my son's innocence. I didn't need any postponements.

Along with all of the above, something else nasty was brewing. About three weeks before the trial, my husband who was still in Canada and had not had the chance to go to Bolivia to liquidate the partnership yet, received a startling phone call from Elizabeth Grontier, our attorney. The legal aid lawyer never gave John Paul or I any insight of the awful and uncanny demand she was presenting to my husband. We would only learn about it later.

The attorney bluntly had said to John, "Mr. Arthur, your wife's and son's trial is been set for October 13, but unless the amount owing to me is paid in full immediately, I will have it indefinitely postponed." A small portion of her fee was still outstanding, but it was the last thing John expected to hear from the lawyer. He was well aware the money owing was rightfully hers, also the financial obligation to *Maitre* Portiere; both, had balances pending. John had explained to the attorneys that as soon as the money from the sale of our house in Bolivia was in his hands, he would immediately wire it to them.

Elizabeth's inexcusable coercion put John between the sword and the spade. Afraid she would execute her threat, he was forced to borrow more money at a super high interest rate. Her action and words could be something a low class blackmailer would do, but not an attorney at law. It was the last straw. From then on, we truly didn't know what else to expect from the French judicial system.

OCTOBER 13, 1986

RESTLESS BUT HOPEFUL WE WAITED FOR THE DAUNTING DATE, October 13th. Undoubtedly the time crawled, but we were sure the end of the tunnel was near. So every Thursday, it was easy for John Paul and I to go over our plans for the future.

After much resistance, J. P. had accepted not to wait for me in France. He would go directly to Canada, where with his Dad's help he would obtain the medical assistance he needed. Thankfully his health had not changed, and with the Lord's blessing and the treatment John Paul will be alright again. It felt good to be able to plan again. Have something as tangible as the trial date helped us dream once more of picking up the pieces and getting on with our lives.

Though it was not easy to stop thinking about the unethical attitude of Elizabeth Grontier, it had left us in a frantic state. The woman knew exactly where she could harm us the most, postponing the trial. My husband just as anxious as us to close the incident in France managed to meet her ruthless demand. At the time he had no idea that her disgraceful threat was just a bluff, impracticable even in France, but what did John or us know about French laws anyway? Our experience with the District Attorney was enough to make us believe anything was possible.

About my surgery, it took place October 9th, in the nick of time. Carried out in one of the city's hospitals, it would be something else I would never forget. Likely my air of grandeur still had a strong hold on me and I needed to go through the awful experience to lose it for good.

As I regained consciousness, I woke up hurting a lot and unable to move even an inch. The anesthesia was wearing off and I realized that I was handcuffed to the hospital bed! Then of all things, I had to go to the bathroom. The officer in charge of my surveillance, male of course, released the manacles that had pinned me to the bed, but only to transfer one to his wrist. Once we reached the spot, he gave me no privacy, this went on until a day later when I was discharged from the hospital and back to prison.

The lump removed from my breast was not life threatening. Yet from the experience I got another life lesson, I became insensitive to anything concerning myself.

In all this time we never heard if the investigation carried out by Interpol was over, or if it was even conducted at all. John Paul and I had our qualms, since no apology came from anyone and the silence made us wonder what else could be in store for us. Elizabeth Grontier was out of the picture, so the only one pleading on our behalf at the Court of Grasse would be *Maitre* Portiere and we didn't even know where we stood with him.

As soon as we learned the date for the trial, I asked Patricia the social assistant to have my husband informed through the Canadian officials in Marseille. It was only fair he received the news as quickly as possible, he was just as anxious as us and by mail it could take forever to reach him.

John subsequently contacted Mrs. Helen Campbell, the Consul in Paris, who now alerted of the date, set my husband's mind at ease. The Consul assured him she would be present at the Court of Grasse on that day. However only as a by-stander. Canadian authorities could not intervene in French judicial matters, but one of their implicit mandates was to give conscious attention to detained Canadian citizens. Information that now came back to us by a letter from my husband sent through the consulate in Marseille.

At 10 o'clock that morning, Judith, John Paul and I were at the Court of Grasse and escorted to the accused's bench. My son sat next to me and we were greatly impressed when the Canadian Consul approached us. True to her word, she was present and wanted to make us aware of her presence in an indeed noble support, even if silent.

Inquisitively our gaze went about the lay out of the place and surprised by the large crowd, I commented with my son, "I don't understand why there are so many people. Those three men dressed in black, with ruffles in their white shirts, facing us; do you think they are the judges? I thought there was only going to be one." John Paul nodded and made me notice something else, "Do you see where the D.A. is seated? There are about ten or more men next to him. I wonder who they are?" We had no chance to say anything else, because the show began.

Maitre Portiere, on our behalf, and *Maitre* Thibault, on Judith's, gave excellent opening statements. For the first time, we heard *Maitre* Portiere expound on our case and defend us with passion. He presented to the court the true tragedy involving my offense, but something unprecedented was taking place.

At first we had no idea what was happening, but we soon found out. The men who sat next to Clavier were also Prosecutors, representatives from all of Southern France. At random they had selected this particular day to be present at this trial in order to set a precedent!

The opening lecture from the delegated Prosecutor was merciless. It negated totally the defense presented by our lawyers. In the dissertation, I was shown as an unscrupulous person. "This woman, from upper middle class, well educated, who in the pursuit of the mighty dollar has used a friend and her son as accomplices to spread a trafficking web to attain material gains."

The accusing words of the delegate were dreadful and he continued with more, "If this hideous gang hadn't been stopped as they were, they would have caused enormous destruction among the French nationals. Their intent was to flood Cannes with Bolivian cocaine!" The speech went even further, "To escape from the rigorous eyes of Justice, they concocted the story that the son of this woman was ill. Your honor, you can see for yourselves that he looks and he is, as healthy as a strong bull."

The attack didn't stop, it continued, "We have to thank the efficiency of the Police Authorities in Perpignan who acted accordingly and prevented drug racketeers from carrying on their damaging as well as elicit trade." Without any interruptions he went ahead and demanded, "These people need to be severely punished so that in the future no one would dare to think that France would tolerate drug traffickers in French territory."

In disbelief the three of us listened to the condemning words. The whole objective was very clear now. It didn't matter to them, who the offenders were, or their circumstances. All the Prosecutors wanted, was to set a precedent against drug lawbreakers who dared smuggle drugs into this part of French territory and we happened to be their scapegoats.

After what took place in that speech, we might as well have been convicted and sentenced before the trial even started; our fate had been sealed. This was not a too far-fetched a possibility, in view of the attitude displayed by the three men of the Tribunal who effectively acted not only as judges but also as jury and all through the delegated prosecutor's opening speech their attention was captured by his verbal rhetoric.

Not so immediately after, a complete lack of interest was shown despite the strong mediation of our respective attorneys, even as each one of us took the stand to present our defense. Their indifference was highly evident, since the judges not only talked among themselves, but because something funny was said they laughed loudly. This impressed on us that they were more concerned in their own private jokes than in what was taking place at the court. It seemed as if our trial was just a parody for them.

Unfortunately at that point our attorneys' intervention no longer seemed to have any purpose.

I still could not dismiss the thought that certainly these men who held justice in their hands would have the ability to differentiate between the chronic offenders the prosecutors had presented us to be, and who we truly were. I also still held the hope that the delegated prosecutor's speech wouldn't completely dissuade the tribunal of my son's innocence.

Throughout the trial the three of us sat in a row, the lawyers on another bench at some distance from us. John Paul, who was next to me, with more insight as to what was to follow, held my hand firmly to give me courage. Once all the expositions were over, we were ordered to stand up as the verdict was pronounced.

"You are all found guilty; each sentenced to ten years in prison!"

Every word seemed to come from another dimension. It was as I had left my body and I was looking down at the scene from afar. In a blur, my eyes misty with tears, I observed my son, the court, and the lawyers, while my body felt almost ready to collapse as I listened to the verdict.

John Paul's life already condemned by a terminal illness, now because of all the blunders that his mother made and the blindness of these so-called judges, he could end up dying imprisoned. AIDS had a survival rate, in the best of circumstances, of two years.

What were these people doing to us? I had been ready to cope with my own chastisement; I was the architect of the affair and deserved the punishment, but John Paul, who never took part in the plot, was convicted just the same. It was in my son's sentencing where the injustice lay.

If a hurricane had swept through, it would have been less devastating than the sentencing, impossible to fathom the reason for so great of a measure of punishment. The blow was too powerful. Had it not been for John Paul who noticed I was about to faint and transferred his grip to my arm, I would have dropped to the floor.

The delegated prosecutor speaker had no right to brand us as an unscrupulous ring of drug racketeers, or to display my action as an elaborated plan to obtain fringe benefits. Instead of the act of a desperate mother, which was the actual fact, no matter how strong a precedent they wanted to set.

If my plan was to swamp the French Riviera with Bolivian cocaine, where were all my contacts? If it was a ring I directed, why had no one else been arrested? Everything was untrue and preposterous.

The District Attorney had built the case against us supported by circumstantial evidence, centered on the information given by the paid informant, Judith's friend. I had no doubt about it now. He chose to ignore my son's innocence, the D.A. paid no heed to my son's HIV diagnosis; strong points that in a less bias court should have exonerated John Paul. Instead, the three men judging us, influenced by the prosecutor's tale, substantiated by the case the District Attorned had built against us, disregarded it.

Everything was too unjust! My rage was not directed only to the judges and the District Attorney; it included our lawyers. I still don't know if the documents and the testimonial letters sent from Bolivia in reference to the integrity of our lives prior to my offense were ever presented. These were important pieces of evidence, but according to the Grontier woman, the District Attorney had not been aware of their existence, and now during this audition, I didn't see or hear *Maitre* Portiere resort to them for his notorious 'surprise move' either.

All that I'd hoped for vanished. Defeated, I was unable to contain the tears of helplessness that now flowed freely down my cheeks.

John Paul seeing my distress, harshly said, "Don't you dare cry now, Mother. Don't give these bastards' satisfaction. Don't you see their contempt? They think we are garbage; *basura Mama*, don't ever do that again. Not while we are here, anyway." My son was right. Even if I was demolished, I had to fight back my frustration and tears.

Seconds later, J. P. gently added, "Mom, please don't cry. God knows the truth. He will find a way to help us out of this mess." I remembered my son saying something similar a few months before. It seemed so long ago now. Yet, he still stood firm that God would find a way out for us.

I suppose countries have their own code of laws to judge and condemn people at fault, but what happened at the trial had not been fair for any one of us, not in accordance to their own standard of law, anyway. We knew of other cases where repeat offenders were handed sentences less harsh than the ones given to us, and we had no previous criminal background. In fact everything that happened at the trial was so cruel that it was even commented on by the media the next day.

The Canadian Consul's presence had been a reassuring sight. At least someone other than us had witnessed what had taken place, even if it was impossible for Canadian authorities to intervene in French judicial affairs.

Before we were taken back to prison, the consul empathetically told us, "I will immediately contact Mr. Arthur. I understand he is waiting anxiously to hear the result of the trial. I'm sorry the news won't be what he expected to hear." Subsequent to what we experienced at the trial, her concern was comforting.

Portiere and Thibault, both attorneys also approached us. They looked as perturbed as we were and in short tried to explain, "The sentencing was so harsh basically because of a fluke: the massive presence of the Prosecutors from Southern France. Portiere even went as far as to say, "I'm positive that if your offense would have remained in the jurisdiction of Perpignan or Marseille, all of you would have been freed by now."

Maitre Portiere, supported by Judith's attorney, put on a fighting front now. "We do have the chance to set things straight," he said, with that phlegmatic smile that I knew so well and which I'd started to despise, "You must file for an appeal. I guarantee the result will be overturned at the Court of Appeals in Aix-en-Provence." His statement made sense, somewhere, someplace, people in charge of justice necessarily would see the perpetrated injustice.

"The preceding trial will be counted as a mistrial, I'm sure," he continued and I believed him. All he said were true facts. The lawyers' conviction set the gears in motion. Back in prison, everyone, social workers, guards as well as inmates encouraged us to follow our attorneys' advice. At the same time we were forewarned the Appeal represented a transfer to a top-security prison in Marseilles, one of the toughest in France! It didn't make any difference. We couldn't just stay at a standstill with such an unjust verdict; all three of us signed the forms.

Soon John Paul's positive thinking was par again, and some hope returned to our hearts. Still, what we experienced at the trial was too brutal to be ignored and we quivered with the thought of the transfer to Marseille. Apparently an extended stay waited for us before our petition for the appeal was even accepted.

The international port in Marseilles was known as a door to the Middle East. It was open to every breed of crime: contraband, drugs, guns and white trade. Therefore the prison's toughness, was parallel to the crimes of the imprisoned subjects. We had A new nightmarish situation ahead of us, but what other choice did we have? None!

My son's resilience to cope with every hindrance we encountered was more than just an inspiration; he was the rock that supported me in my weakest moments. Paradoxically at this point, la *maison* became an even stronger hold of safety for us, thanks to the astonishing understanding we had found in guards and prisoners; unfortunately it was soon to be lost.

Even my walk back to the Lord was threatened. I was contending with an extremely powerful enemy: doubt! Depressed and angry, I asked Him, "Whatever happened to my prayers Lord?" All I heard back were the words pronounced at the trial, "You are all sentenced to ten years in prison!" So, where was the God that let this happen?

Fray Regis tried his mightiest to make me understand that all that I was experiencing was transient and that one day the purpose of this journey would become very clear to me. I wondered when, if ever.

The Canadian Consul was the one to give my husband the blow. At a great distance away, our son's ailment became his biggest concern. John, who was just as convinced as us that John Paul would have a favorable verdict, could not comprehend the injustice done to him, nor the severity of the sentencing for all. John's situation in Canada was not the best either. He was economically stressed, but my husband's supportive letters never stop coming, neither did Patrick's. Both continued to be a strong source of encouragement.

John Paul's endurance was admirable. I would have liked to have it myself. In one of my depressed moments, I remembered so clearly when he told me, "Mother, the result of this trial shouldn't shake our faith in God. I believe all that has happened and is still going to happen is part of the required growing process we need to go through. Mistakes have to be rectified, so that we can reach the spiritual maturity our Supreme Creator expects from us."

My son's words impacted me. I wasn't sure if I should now feel greater shame for the situation I created, or feel blessed. Had I not been incarcerated, my values would have never come back to me; I was blessed in that sense. If I hadn't lost my values in the first place, prison would have never happened. It was a riddle all right. Rev. Fray Regis had been so right about men, not being as compassionate and forgiving as our Lord.

The Fray's presence during my time in Nice was another source of strength. Without his guidance, I know, my spiritual warfare would have been a lot tougher. He helped me better understand the Holy Scriptures. The Letters from *Paul* touched me the deepest, the slight similitude of our situations perhaps? He had been imprisoned for being righteous, me for doing the opposite, but imprisoned just the same!

November 10, 1986

Alerted of the violence and trickery running rampant at *Des Baumettes*, the Marseille's prison, we knew the road ahead would be difficult and naturally dreaded the transfer. Four days after his 26th birthday, John Paul was the first to be transferred; I learned the news through the short letter he wrote.

November 10th 1986,

Dear Mom,

This is a quick one. I don't have much time; I have just been notified and ordered to pack my belongings. I'm leaving for Marseille in a couple of hours. We will probably see each other once you transfer too. I'm well and happy because this will put us one step closer to home.

Look after yourself. I love you Mom, J. P

This letter was the last I would receive from my son for a long while and I withered with worry. I tried to placate my concern in different ways, but mainly praying. Pleading with God to keep John Paul well and to make my transfer imminent, I didn't care if that prison was the world's worst. If John Paul was there, likely going through hell, I didn't see why I should be spared.

Judith's transfer and mine came through a week before Christmas. Just before leaving *La Maison*, the Warden requested our presence in her office. This was a bit unusual, but she wanted us to know she was sending a special letter to the prison's authorities in Marseille, where apparently the Warden made reference to our good behavior while in Nice. She then personally oversaw that the letter was enclosed in the manila envelope, together with the rest of our files; documents that would be taken to Marseilles by the police in charge of our custody. As a farewell the Warden was allowing us to witness the more humane side of her personality.

Our relocation took place in a Police Patrol vehicle. No humiliating looks from any by-passers, or screeching sirens, or mobilized police escorts followed us. I can honestly say that except for the handcuffs, we received fair treatment during the two-hour drive; but from what we had heard, what waited for us at *Des Baumettes* was terrifying!

Nothing even came close to what we actually faced. We arrived at about 8 a.m. on a Saturday, which apparently complicated matters. The guards on duty, who were few, had neither the time nor the obligation to review the files of inmates transferred on a weekend. The letter from the Warden and documents sent from Nice remained unopened and probably locked in a drawer.

The personnel simply followed the customary weekend routine for new arrivals and Judith and I were placed in a cell on the ground floor, a section where only troublemakers and high-security inmates were kept, and the cell's sole occupant, proved to be a threat to our safety!

The moment the door shut, she began to throw everything within her reach against the walls. Swearing profanities and giving us menacing looks she screamed, "I don't want anyone here. You better get these bitches out of my cell or I will make sure someone is hurt! You will be sorry." All the forewarnings about the place were overshadowed by our present reality.

The racket brought back the two guards who likely afraid for our safety removed us from that cell and placed us in another. The two inmates in this one didn't look too friendly either. They were heavy built and spoke in an unintelligible language, perhaps Arabic; in Nice, we were told a large percentage of *Des Baumettes'* population came from Tunisia, Algiers, or Morocco. At least these two didn't toss things around or try to harm us. But by now, terrified and on the verge of tears, Judith and I didn't dare move or say anything.

While we were still in that state, a guard came to rescue us, but it was only to let us out for the morning promenade. Most inmates were already out, so it was just us walking behind the guard. As we stepped outside the building, the rescue feeling vanished and was replaced by the disheartening sight we had in front of us. First we passed a solid stonewall, broke only by a small barred gate where several inmates stood watching us. We recognized a couple from Nice. The enclosure behind the wall seemed large, had dirt ground, no plants and looked ugly. Ugly or not, it was not the designated area for us.

Walking a few more meters and the area we left behind seemed like a Garden of Eden compared to the two enclosed spaces we now had in our view. Each of about two hundred square feet, one next to the other, a high stonewall surrounded the whole section, crowned by rows of barbed wire. A metal grill separated the two, which extended to the top, as a lid, converting the two pens into actual cages.

My friend and I had not stopped shaking from what we had experienced moments before and we now had to deal with this new shocking situation. As we stepped inside one of the partitions, the fourteen inmates in the interior displayed a bellicose attitude, but didn't touch us. Of course not, how could they? We looked like just two little scared mice unable to fend for ourselves.

Our first promenade at *Des Baumettes* was overwhelming to say the least. Warily my heart shrunk as I wondered, "If Judith and I are going through such appalling experiences, what must my son's situation be like?"

Once the outing was over the guards got everyone back to their cells; as we entered the one assigned to us, we were told, "Pick up your belongings, you are coming with us." It appeared that as an afterthought they had changed their original view and decisively reviewed our files. Reading the recommendations given by the Warden in Nice and on their own accord the custodians decided to move us to the second floor. The humane act of the Warden had saved us!

The difference we found was quite obvious, not an awful lot in appearance but we appreciated the quietness, especially after the downstairs' havoc. Our walk ended in front of the last door on the left of the hallway. Once inside, we found no extreme variations from the cell we had in Nice. Except for the two bunk beds at opposite sides and by the look of things the lower ones were taken; the two occupants who appeared to be French unhurriedly got up from the cots to great us. "I am Chantal and this is Luciane. You can have the top bunks," one of them said.

Their manner was civilized, we appreciated that much, but I had never slept in a bunk bed, let alone on the upper part of one. I was a bit leery about my capabilities of sleeping higher up, better say, I was afraid I might roll over on the floor, but I knew I had to do it no matter what. So I climbed the four steps up the steel narrow ladder, to leave a handful of personal things and actually it didn't feel bad considering that in Nice all I had was a mattress on the floor.

After we finished accommodating our stuff, Chantal who seemed the talkative one filled us with some of the *Des Baumettes'* history. It appears that German Nazis and their French collaborators built it during the Second World War. At the time it served to imprison war prisoners, but presently the only lodgers were convicted criminals and from the little Judith and I experienced at

des Baumettes to this point, it lived up to its past and present reputation; enough to make us quiver. Our permanence in Marseille
was going to be tougher than what we had anticipated and we did
not even have an idea when our appeal would take place.

It was a lot to assimilate in our first day at Des Baumettes, but
Chantal's next words caught my full attention, "The buildings
next to ours are part of the men's Penitentiary.

Sometimes using a small mirror I sneak a quick look and
observe what is going on over there, even if all I'm able to see are
the inmate's hands stretching out through the bars, or discarding
refuse." The topic was more than interesting for me. My son had
to be in one of those buildings, I had to investigate further. So I
asked Chantal to lend me the mirror. She didn't object, instead I
was shown how the spying was done.

Stepping on the chair placed under the window, I stretched out
my arm through the bars; my eyes focus on the mirror that once
it was positioned the way Chantal explained, the reflection of the
edifices should come in my view. My attempt paid off, I saw the
two large buildings she mentioned, one after the other and next
to ours, obviously part of the men's quarters.

The structures were four stories high, with numerous windows,
likely barred too and I could not make out exactly how many. The
rectangular mirror that I used as a periscope didn't have the range
to be that accurate, but I counted at least sixty on every floor. I
supposed one window per cell the same as in our building and
who knows how many inmates in each, since *Des Baumettes* was
the largest prison in all Southern France.

For unknown reasons, male prisoners discarded their waste
chucking it through the windows and the refuse landed into an
approximate twelve feet area through out the long stretch of
the buildings. Supposedly at one time that space was a security
feature that separated the buildings from the massive perim-
eter wall. Except that now thanks to the unorthodox method of
garbage disposal, it looked more like a compost pit.

The material left decaying for long periods of time, surely would become a health threat for the overcrowded inmate population. Infectious diseases could bread and multiplied, while insects would do the rest, for what could have been easily prevented. Most disgraceful considering that France was not an underdeveloped country.

Des Baumettes is still in use to this day and from present broadcasting news the conditions had not improved, but worsened instead, if that could be possible!

Some days later I realized that all that filth necessarily had to compromise the meal preparation, which the same as in Nice was prepared at the men's side; the cockroaches, hairs, and other stuff we found floating in the coffee and in most of the daily courses was enough evidence to attest to it. More than disgusting, however if you had enough money you could find a quick remedy to the problem; order better meals through the canteen, hypothetically prepared somewhat in more hygienic conditions.

With hardly nothing to do in the cell, it seemed that it was a common practiceg to listen to cellmates' felony accounts here too. So in no time we learned a lot about our roommates, like Luciene, she mentioned to have been a *Madame;* women who owned or ran a bawdy house were known by that term. She had been engaged in this illegal activity, and even if the trade had been around from the beginning of time and running strong in France, it was still an outlaw pursuit and the reason for Luciene's imprisonment.

While Chantal who also shared the reasons of her incarceration simply saying, "I'm here serving two years sentence for drug trafficking. I was in the process of selling ten pounds of hashish, when I got caught."

Then Christmas arrived and we were inside the least likely of places I would have ever dreamed to be, *Des Baumettes* in Marseilles, and I still had no news from my son. In five more days, a whole year would have gone by since the day we were arrested. Thirty-six days from the time I received John Paul's last letter and almost the same amount of days, since I last saw him.

Sixty-eight days since we had been condemned and I begun to feel buried alive!

During the same time, two years prior, we were still a happy family; nothing much troubled us except for the rampant inflation our country was going through. John Paul had just returned from California to spend Christmas at home and in keeping with the family tradition, we all went to the midnight mass, my mother included. After the service we had a late supper and later we opened up presents.

Then last year, because John and Patrick planned to spend Christmas with his parents in Canada, we commemorated the festivity a few days earlier; even opened a few presents. Except that this time the celebration was not as meaningful for John Paul or I; the affliction of the illness dug already deep into our hearts.

Now at the vigil of Christmas, I could not have been more depressed as I reminisced on the past, until at 5 p.m. something unexpected came to lift up my spirit. Together with the meal of the day, I received several letters from my son, as well as two from Canada and one from Bolivia. I could not have wished for better Christmas presents and the best one was to learn that John Paul was fine. The timing was extraordinary!

More Christmas surprises streamed in the next morning, when the cell opened and one of the guards announced, "In half and hour, Fray Charles the Catholic Chaplain will come to celebrate Mass for inmates who wish to attend. I'll be back a few minutes before that time to summon any one who wants to participate; each should bring out their own chair."

It was great to learn that even at des Baumettes, such a startling event, the birth of our Lord Jesus was celebrated with the service of the Holy Mass. As the guard stated, just before 10 a.m. our cell was open and the four of us went out with our respective chairs.

At one end of the hallway, a table covered with the customary white tablecloth and a stand with a Crucifix in the middle, was set as an improvised altar; the chairs were placed in rows of six. Most inmates participated, but not all were Catholics, their nasty behavior gave them away, though they calmed down once the priest arrived. The reason for such a large turn over was because a number of those women had been at *Les Baumettes* in previous Christmas, and knew about the treat that followed right after Mass. The Catholic Church provided an out of the ordinary breakfast, which included hot chocolate, cheese and croissants.

Once the service concluded I had the opportunity to speak with the priest, who when he learned my son was also incarcerated, made my day saying, "Later I will celebrate Mass at the men's side. I will make sure John Paul is called for the service." The priest's words cheered me up. It would be great for John Paul to join in the celebration; he would also have something positive to entertain his thoughts and perhaps a good breakfast as well.

Understanding that father Charlie regularly visited inmates who requested it, I asked him, "Would it be possible for you to come and visit us?" His response, though negative brought another alternative. "I'm swarmed with work and requests. I'm sorry; I don't have any time to spare. However if you speak Spanish, I could refer you to another Catholic priest, the Rev. Fray Jacques Montes. He volunteers his visits for Spanish speaking inmates. Would you be interested in seeing him, instead?"

"Yes of course, I would be very happy." I answered and he promised to look into it and continued with his rounds.

As soon as the bureaucratic machine at *Des Baumettes* got rolling, the visiting privileges my son and I had in Nice got also re-established. But here it took place only every other week, and even if the time was doubled, it was more of a setback for me. It was best when weekly I could verify with my own eyes if John Paul was well; but it was something else among other things that my son and I would need to adjust to.

The morning of the prescribed day, after the stripping and searching process, we didn't just walk to our destination, the same as in Nice. Here we boarded a small buss with barred windows, and well guarded we were driven to the males' prison, even if it was just around the corner.

The minute the bus stopped, we were ordered to disembark and directed to the visitation site. No surprises here, the security glass built-in on one of the walls separating the visitors, was in place. Even so I was able to appreciate that my son looked alright, but I had to ask him anyway, "How are you John Paul; how is your health holding on? I know the conditions here are awful, how are you coping?"

"I'm fine, Mom. Of course the place is a lot worse than *la maison*, but I'm managing. I already have a job, which keeps me busy. I draw characters for the prison's journal. The reference letters my teacher and the Warden from Nice wrote helped me a lot. I'm actually treated quite fairly." My son told me smiling and not stressed, which helped set my mind at ease.

John Paul with something else in his mind continued, "From my window I can see some of the women's buildings. So now Mom, I need to know where your cell is situated. Is it facing south or north? If its south, you should be able to see the sun going up in the morning and going down late in the afternoon; mine faces that way and it's the fourth window on the third floor in the building next to the females'." As he waited for my reply, J. P. had a mischievous glare in his eyes.

It took me a couple of minutes to position myself versus his cell. Once I had it, I responded, "Mine is the last one on the second floor, in the building neighboring yours." With this established and since both our cells faced south, J.P. figured we were less than one hundred feet apart and even in Marseille my son's resourcefulness found us an unauthorized way to communicate with each other.

As soon as we were back in our respective cells, after some maneuvering we managed to distinguish each other's window. This was a balancing act for me, considering that I stood on the back of a chair, clenched onto the window bars with one hand, while I held the mirror, my periscope tool in the other and with the only purpose to jest greeting to my son across cyber space, all the while hoping not to fall or get caught.

A week or two later, we even figured that this form of contact with the help of the Morse code that John Paul sent in a letter to refresh my memory, it could serve to convey important delayed news not included in our daily letters.

We used colored garments to send the coded messages, white for the dots, scarlet for the lines, yellow after each letter and green to end the word. Judith, Chantal or Luciene, helped. I red out loud the colors, one of the girls wrote them down, and later I interpreted the colors writing down the corresponding symbols. Per example scarlet, white, scarlet yellow, scarlet, scarlet, scarlet, yellow, white, white, white, scarlet, yellow, white, yellow, green. Scarlet, white, scarlet, scarlet, yellow, scarlet, scarlet, scarlet, yellow, white, white, scarlet, green; would read, Love You.

Quite a puzzle and at first deciphering the messages was like riding on a turtle's back, very slow, but with practice we managed to do it like in the good old days, when the telegraph was the only fast method of communication. Childish again, but it had an adventurous flare and a way to escape from our real environment. The same as in Nice, it gave us the feeling of having some control over our lives and a breath of freedom in play-land.

Then came the visits of Father Juan Montes. Referred by the chaplain, he visited both Judith and I, but separately. Inspired by his cordiality and title, I opened up to him immediately. For the first time in more than a year, I was able to tell this priest everything, my entire Calvary from beginning to end and in my own language. Father Juan, understanding my pain, gave a lot of himself to console me and right after our visit he went to see John Paul.

A few sessions later we nominated Father Montes our Champion; vanquisher of the three. Born in Barcelona, Spain, he brought not only the joy of his presence, but also the pleasure of listening my language, Spanish. He became our friend; more like a Guardian Angel during the stormy time at *Des Baumettes*. On several occasions Rev. Juan even called my husband on our behalf, giving him more recent news about our situation. This helped to ease John's mind.

Once we were moved to the second floor, the improvement also extended to the promenade. The outings were in the one where we saw the girls from Nice, no grilled cages here. Fridays and Saturdays in the afternoon, a man and a woman who were physical educators came to make us practice some exercises and other times to play volleyball games.

These outings were not mandatory, only inmates who freely wanted to participate were called out. Judith and I never failed to go. Actually we enjoyed ourselves while in the games. It would not be long before the P.E.s became our friends too.

Early in January, Judith and I obtained a job doing piecework brought to the prison by entrepreneurs from outside. The hourly remuneration was far more than what I had earned in Nice; this unexpected gain could not have come in a better timing. John was still without a job. The little left from the sale of our unfinished house was almost depleted and there was no certainty when the rest of our assets would be liquidated.

It was good that John Paul and I worked. The Francs we received went to pay for the special canteen orders; we just couldn't handle the daily meals served by the prison; there were too many bugs, dead or alive, battling for the servings!

While in Canada, even Patrick who throughout his entire young life had people around serving him, grasping the family's financial distress found work in a burger place. He worked every day after school. His earnings gave him spending money for his personal needs. Everyone in my family had responded to my *affair* only with love and support.

My mother who acted as my husband's proxy had gone out of her way to procure the sale of our beautiful but unfinished house. Unfortunately for the assets owned in partnership with Mauricio, John had to be in Bolivia to dissolve the businesses and sale the part corresponding to us, but he was still in Quesnel.

As important as it was his return trip, it was postponed several times. Sure of the promises made by our lawyers, John remained in Canada; he wanted to be available for the moment John Paul was set free. The trial was over and our son was in Marseille instead of heading for Canada, so I expected to hear from my husband, notifying us he was on his way to Bolivia.

In the mist of this endless stack of tribulations, a ray of sunshine tiptoed inside the prison walls. An extraordinary person came into John Paul's life. Regina Castang, a doctor in medicine, who out of the goodness of her heart visited prisoners as a volunteer. She somehow connected with my son and periodically visited him. J. P. had then the opportunity to talk with her privately and in depth on the subject of his illness. For the first time since his arrival to France, John Paul received invaluable information about AIDS from this unselfish scientist.

The moment I was granted permission from the warden, the doctor extended her visits to me too and I saw Regina as often as John Paul. She was one of the kindest people I ever met in France and the second Guardian Angel we found in Marseilles. Patiently as only true angels have, Regina shed light on my ignorance of AIDS.

She carefully explained what exactly meant to be HIV positive and in which way this virus would affect my son's life. Since I still had big lapses with French, she spoke in English and thanks to her, I came to understand the difference between being HIV positive and having AIDS per say. "Just because John Paul has been tested HIV positive, doesn't mean he has what is known as full-blown AIDS, or that he will soon die," Regina said making sure I understood every word before she continued.

"We know of HIV cases that have carried the virus for eight years, perhaps some even more. Scientists are trying to prove that the survival time rate could be longer. This position is still under investigation because AIDS as an epidemic is so recent." This conversation took place at beginning of 1987, when HIV and AIDS were pretty much in nebulous for the general public.

Regina continued lecturing me on other important views on the virus, "When the affected person's immune system is weakened to the point that it's impossible to fight new ailments, then and only then, is the person diagnosed as having full-blown AIDS." Quietly Regina looked at me to see if I had assimilated her words. Satisfied, she added, "AIDS is not the killing agent Myriam; death occurs because of the other ailments."

It was only after her explanations that I was able to understand what to expect from this virus. However, even with that small light of hope she had brought to me, it still meant a delayed death sentence on my son's life, which only a miracle could change. Nonetheless, it was uplifting to at least know that while my son's blood count remained where it was, there was no chance of an immediate death.

Only through her recommendation and help it was that the prison's doctor checked John Paul regularly, and some weeks later by a renowned specialist. Regina advised J.P. to keep a well-balanced diet, to help build up and sustain his immune system, something that while in Nice intuitively I had asked John Paul to do. Now with the accurate facts presented by our new friend, John Paul made sure to supplement at Des Baumettes too.

While John was in Canada, had not crossed his arms either. Right after he was notified of the devastating result of our trial, my husband became aware of an existing agreement between the French and Canadian Governments for a possible exchange of inmates. At once he contacted the department of Foreign Affairs in Ottawa and learned that the accord enable prisoners serve their sentences in their home country, with the intent of bringing families together.

My husband immediately tried to initiate the procedures for our transfer to Canada. To his dismay he learned an immediate relocation was not possible. Established rules first had to be complied with, such as that all processes be concluded before a transfer would even be considered; ours was far from being closed for the reason of the appeal. Consequently we were bound to Marseilles until our case was fully closed.

In the meantime Mrs. Campbell, the Canadian Consul, through proper channels made accessible to John Paul and I explicit material regarding the possible transfer. She sent booklets with information relevant to the Correctional System and Parole Board in Canada, a copy for each; documents that my son and I avidly read and compared thoughts on in our bi-weekly visits. The information reflected that everything would be far better in Canada than what awaited for us in France.

Seeing all that material and understanding what could come out from it, Judith's curious requested, "Do you think the Canadian Consul could inquire on my behalf whether a similar agreement exists between the United States and France? I've dual citizenship, American and French. If it exists, I would like to be transferred to the States to serve my sentence close to my children. They reside in Minneapolis now under the care of my sister Martha."

The consul kindly accepted the task and after contacting the American Consulate found the information Judith needed. The answer was affirmative. Judith could also benefit from such a transfer. My friend then asked her family to get detail information from the United States Government on the required stipulations for such a transfer to take place.

While John in Canada, in constant contact with the Canadian Authorities learned that there was not much else he could do to expedite our transfer and since his trip to Bolivia could not be postponed any longer, my husband left for my country January 11th, 1987.

Leaving our son Patrick, who had just turned 16, entrusted with a Power of Attorney and instructions to deposit the checks John expected to send from the proceeds of the partnership's dissolution; they had jointly opened a bank account for that purpose and Patrick was also to remain attentive to any communication from the Ministry of Foreign Affairs, making sure that what ever was needed from that office, or by us, was immediately taking care off.

My husband never mentioned it, but I was certain that his trip back to my country necessarily had to be a dreaded nightmare. After a year of what happened in France, John would face friends, relatives and withstand the embarrassment of their questioning. I was also sure he would never say anything about our son's ailment, while at the same time he would not allow anyone to utter negative remarks about me. I could not but admired my husband for his courage and respected him even more for it.

He anticipated that the dissolution and subsequent sale of our assets, would not take more than a month or two at the most, so John planned to stay in Bolivia only the necessary time. Except that the Bolivian economy had actually worsened, inflation was as rampant and money was just as scarcer as before. Our partner was having more than enough problems just trying to keep the factory afloat, which made the separation of the partnership extremely difficult.

It took weeks of negotiations for my husband and Mauricio to reach an agreement whereby all the shares John and I had in the factory were transferred to our partner and his wife. In exchange, my husband took title of the remaining real estate properties owned by the firm: the house we were living in, and the parcel of land intended for a subdivision, disregarding that the value of those properties was less than one third the value of the factory.

Not too favorable solution, but in reality it was the only possible option and John consented hoping that the assets would sale quickly. Yet in spite that he had lowered the prices to a bare minimum, there were no offers; the real estate market unfortunately was as good as dead.

While John was experiencing only disappointments and frustration in Bolivia, Judith's family in America, alarmed with the ten-year sentence their sister received, decided to engage the services of two new lawyers. *Maitre La Pointe*, a renowned attorney from Paris and Maitre K. Mouret from Marseilles, this last one as a go-between with *La Pointe* and Judith to handle judicial errands.

The siblings were doing the best to assist their sister, within their economical means. All great, but their effort brought more dismay to my heart! Surely my son deserved a better defense in the appeal too; certainly superior than what we experienced with Portiere. Except that to think of hiring another lawyer in my husband's present situation was just out of the question, financial matters would become even more difficult for him. It had not been too long ago that the balance owing to *Maitre* was finally paid.

But much was at stake for our son, so I wrote to John anyway so we could consult on the subject together. Sometimes I believe God puts us to the test, but while doing so, He also opens amazing avenues of hope, such as when my mother, who now realizing the gravity of our situation, our sentences, my husband's lack of money, and wanting to help, put my father's bequest estate to her up for sale.

The Spanish style house where my sister and I grew up, and where my parents and us, as a family had memorable memories. Dad designed the layout of the house himself, but had it built by contractors under his supervision; he was already retired from the army and had the time. Centrally located at only a block and a half from the school my sister and I attended, and the St. Claire convent and Church, where mother went for Mass almost every morning

The place had six apartments; five were rental units, built around three large courtyards that had some small fruit trees and many flowery plants, though my parent's favorites were the roses. My mother loved to tend it all and kept the yards manicured.

The first patio at the front was built specifically for parties, it had an Andalusian flair; grape vines, sustained by eight brick pillars painted white and intertwined through the trellises above. Ceramic tiles were on the floor as well as on the benches built against the wall for seating. A fountain in the middle, with the water spraying out from the top of a small replica of the Illimani Andean mountain, my father being from La Paz had to have it. My sister and I had incredible parties here, especially during the Carnival festivity; our father had been very wise in having this recreational area built for our use, it was indestructible!

Now my dearest mother for the reason of my situation had put the place for sale and because the price was right and the property not only was beautiful but also created good revenue, sold quickly; before any of our own properties. I learned later that Mom handed thirty thousand American dollars to John, and an equal amount to my sister, as an advance inheritance to each. She then purchased a comfortable condominium unit in a new building for herself, to which my husband facilitated her move.

Extraordinary sacrifices everyone made: John, my mother now, and even Patrick to help cope with our present circumstances, the aftermath of my transgression. It was impossible not to realize how great their love was, as well as the Lord's that up until then I had taken for granted.

It was at this point that John received my query letter about lawyers and without delay contacted Mrs. Campbell, the Canadian Consul with a fast message, "Will you please let Myriam know that I was dissatisfied with the way Portiere handled the case in Nice. It's important my wife and son have a better defense on the appeal. Alert her that she should contract the services of a new attorney; I'll give instructions to Patrick to wire immediately the required amount to the Consulate in Marseille."

The message was immediately sent to me in a note from the consulate and encouraged by my husband's advice I went ahead and decided to look for a good lawyer for the appeal. Carefully with my son, we reviewed the all facts and arrived to the conclusion that it would be wiser this time, if the three of us would have the same lawyer. Judith also agreed. At once John Paul and I wrote to *Maitre* La Pointe to this effect. His response was immediate; he accepted our case.

Some days later, I received a letter from my husband with complete details about the money my mother so generously had given him. Also telling me his decision to remained in Bolivia. His goal was to stay until all our assets were sold, aiming to recover as much cash as possible from our investments. Vital for our new start in Canada, but regrettably it would take longer than what he had anticipated.

Since *Maitre* La Pointe accepted, *Maitre* Portiere had to be notified; therefore I wrote to him, asking him to collaborate with his colleague from Paris by handing over our dossier together with all the Bolivian and Californian documents my husband had sent.

His response was fast; in his letter the attorney politely indicated that he was not only obligated to collaborate, but also to plead on our behalf. Portiere chose this opportunity to let me know that we still owed him money. He claimed that the original forty five thousand francs he quoted at the beginning of the investigation were still up and running, since it was him who had filed for our appeal. This was the part that Sylvie had left out when she translated Portiere's response about his fees while still in Nice!

It was a perturbing and unexpected charge; I would have happily fired him, but fear of another daunting surprise as the one the Grontier woman had pulled from under her sleeve stopped me; the referral documents were in his hands. Instead, cautiously I wrote back stating that in my understanding his services had been paid in full, but that I would let my husband know of this new demand.

Weeks later, we were notified that March 19, 1987 was the set date for our appeal. From what we were told by our original lawyers, we were confident that in this court our case would have a more favorable reception from the judges, so our expectations could not have been any greater!

Certainly we were more than ready and anxious to face the court, but something else difficult to understand held up the process; we questioned ourselves if we had been jinxed from the start, or what? Otherwise why did we meet head-on with this new obstacle?

The same date our appeal had to take place was assigned for an important trial in Paris, where *Maitre La Point,* our renowned Parisian attorney, was the main defendant. As a result he could not be present in ours. He asked us to sign adjourning papers applying for another date, that is if we still wanted him to act as our attorney. The situation didn't leave us much choice, so we signed.

Then more interruptions kept adding to the pile, it was like a paradox had taken over. No soon the new date was fixed when the two lawyers from Nice; Judith's who had remained as her defendant too and ours, requested another postponement on the appeal's date, this time to June 1$^{st.}$ On their own accord, the two attorneys had engaged the change without even asking us if we would agree to have it amend and there was nothing we could do to stop the action; the notification came by mail, with a copy to Maitre La Pointe.

It was just too much to bear; after more than six months in Marseille, Judith, John Paul, and I were dreadfully worn out, and all we wanted was to be freed from the French judicial system. So to make sure there were not going to be anymore postponements, we wrote to our lawyers, with a copy to the Court of Appeals, giving them all an ultimatum conveying our irrevocable decision to be tried on that date, if necessary without their presence!

We still expected a fair resolution from our plea, but since we already knew the existing flaws in the French judicial structure, it prepared us for whatever the result might be. We now had another form of escape: our transfers!

JUNE 1, 1987

AT LAST ON JUNE 1ST, WE WERE AT THE COURT OF APPEALS IN AIX-en-Province; the appeal took place on the set date. All the lawyers were present, even the renowned one from Paris, but it didn't make any difference. The verdicts virtually did not change; again we were all found guilty. My sentence remained unchanged, 10 years, John Paul's and Judith's were lowered to seven years. In my son's case the injustice prevailed, to a lesser degree in Judith's, but an unfairness just the same.

Was the Judge's decision here bound by the existing claim from the Prosecutors in Grasse? It had to be, otherwise why did he ignore the solid defenses presented by our lawyers? I suppose we would never find out, but it didn't matter anymore, but the comedy was not over yet.

A week later, John Paul, Judith and myself each received letters from the three attorneys, giving us their stern advice to file for another appeal. This time to the Supreme Court in Paris, where according to them we would have a fair trial. John Paul would be acquitted, my sentence reduced to a three years maximum and Judith freed because of the time she'd already served.

When I saw my son in our next scheduled visit, we talked about the suggestion and we plain out laughed! Informed by other sources, we understood that it could take up to two years just to have a date set for an appeal in Paris; not counting all the extra money it would represent. We believed in our lawyers' promises at the trial, trusted their advice for a second round at the appeal, but a third one...definitely not! Judith also agreed.

We found their suggestion preposterous. The attorneys must have thought we continued to be as naïve as before, or perhaps crazy that we would even consider such irrational advice. If the counselors were not there just for the money, they certainly were the ones out of their minds!

It was more important for us now to have the court case closed. So we could start the procedures for our transfers to Canada and the United States, where we would finish the unjust sentences handed over to us, near our families and in far better conditions than what we found in France.

Thankfully John Paul's health had kept well, but in the summer of 1987 the situation in the male sector of *des Baumettes* became unbearable. Riots took place everywhere; fires were set in different areas, one in the vicinity to John Paul's cell. From behind the bars of my window I could see the black smoke coming out from his cell as well as from others nearby, downright dangerous for my son. I panicked with the thought that J.P. could be trapped inside, burned, or suffocated by the smoke.

Doubt and fear surmounted again; it seems that each time I was faced with a new challenge I blamed my creator for it, "What is the matter Lord, why do you keep giving me one trial after another; don't you think I have had enough?"

It's a wonder God didn't give up on me; but no harm came to my son. As a safety measure, when the fire broke out, the guards unlocked cell doors, a contributing factor in increasing the number of rioters, but John Paul had the presence of mind to find a quiet cell far from the fire. He knew the occupants and wisely remained there until the specialized riot platoon got control of the situation.

After such a horrifying experience, it would have been more than insane to listen to our lawyers. What we needed was to leave France as soon as possible.

The Canadian Consul in Paris helped a lot. Not necessarily with the transfer itself, no. It was beyond her influence, but she constantly updated us with news. Her letters became our life support while we waited, but the process ended being more intricate than expected. More procedures had to be fulfilled before the French Authorities would even consider the transfer; such as paying Customs fines and Court fees.

The fines alone represented a very costly disbursement. The government demanded millions of Francs in penalty for the importation. I tried to negotiate for a reduction, but the existing bureaucracy prolonged the wait. We remained in Marseille longer than we ever dreamed possible and or course my guilt escalated.

What had I accomplished other than to put my entire family through horrific and sad experiences? My husband, who was fifty-five years old, had been forced to leave his livelihood behind and give up his renowned professional career in Bolivia on account of what I had done. John and I had worked hard and steady to obtain the financial stability that at one time we enjoyed and now, once again my husband was forced to sell below cost a parcel of land, to meet the French monetary demand.

To see it all go up in smoke hurt me. These were only material losses true, but all were expenditures associated with my transgression, and helped me to open my eyes even more to the greatness of the man I married. Without a thought for himself, or ever a word of reproach, John focused only on getting his son and wife out of France.

Thanks to John's unwavering support, John Paul and I handled our imprisonment much better. We knew the end of the tunnel was near. After the fire, the male sector's condition at *des Baumettes* worsened; consequently it was irresponsible on my part to keep waiting for any reductions. Instead, I authorized the

Canadian Consulate to pay the requested amount made available to us by my husband.

Besides something else compelled my decision; John Paul and I received shattering news from Bolivia. Actually it was my sister, who informed me in a letter, "Your husband's endurance is at a breaking point Myriam! Since his return to Bolivia, John had confronted only negativity." I knew this could happen, but in my own selfish agony, I didn't see the possible consequences.

"Mom called and told me," My sister wrote in her letter. "She is having difficulty coping with John's latest behavior. Alone, in your house in *Aranjuez,* he is drinking heavily. Frustrated and under the influence of alcohol he sometimes uses his gun, shooting bullets in the air to silence barking dogs, disturbing the neighbors."

This was worrisome news, and until then I didn't realize how desperate my husband must have been as he was unable to sell our properties and powerless to do anything to fix our situation in France. I was directly responsible for everything, more so for the change in John's conduct. I knew my husband needed his family intact and near him to overcome the distress, but sadly we were behind bars, helpless. All John Paul and I could do was write to John and lay out optimistic plans for our future, frantically trying to remove our crushing reality from his mind. It was our turn to encourage him.

A few weeks later I received a letter from the Canadian Consul with copy to J.P. It brought altogether reassuring news!

October 29, 1987

"Mr. Arthur has just called and informed me that your house in Aranjuez has been sold. Some of your belongings are being now packaged and shipped by Air-cargo to Canada. Your mother is left in trust of the sales of the other building lots,

so he will fly back to Canada, November 11th. He has asked me to give you the good news.

Yours truly, H. Campbell "

J.P. and I needed the boost. Eight months had gone by after the appeal, three after the fines had been totally paid, but our dossier remained stagnant somewhere, waiting for some missing signatures to close it. In spite of that, the hope that our transfer had to take place sooner or later, kept us going; otherwise we would have gone insane.

We expected the notification any time now, but it was Judith's transfer that took place first. She left for the USA, April 19th, 1988. Her departure was a step forward but left me lonesome. My friend and I had shared our sorrows and every thought that went through our minds for almost two and a half years. I knew she had a difficult trail in front of her; Judith's husband had not been as forgiving as mine. He continued to work abroad, and the few times he came to see her, made sure she fully felt the burden of her fault. As she departed, we both cried and wished each other better times in the life ahead.

Two weeks later, May 3rd my notification arrived, short and concise, "You will be transferred tomorrow to Paris." The guard said without any other information, but my son and I had been alerted by the Canadian Consul and knew the pertinent steps that would follow. "You will go first to Paris, likely together, since you both are scheduled for the International Transfer, but placed in different prisons until the transatlantic flight can be arranged for the departure at an immediate date."

It was so gratifying to see that John Paul was already in the police van that would transport us to Paris. Except that this time he not only was cuffed but shackled too, which was heartbreaking. Likely I was a pitiful sight too, since this time I also wore the infamous bracelets, but not the shackles. As the gates of Les

Baumettes closed behind the van, I though it would great if I could just board-up as easily this episode in our lives, but it was easier said than done!

The consul's forewarning was precise; J. P. and I were separated in Paris and my *adieu* to France in the Parisian prison was overwhelming to say the least. Another incident not too easily to forget waited for me; I happened to share the cell with an inmate who was experiencing agonizing withdrawal addiction signs. When she was not vomiting, she lay almost immobilized on her cot, shivering. Then when nothing seemed to be left in her stomach, she heaved, coughing a pink substance, probably vile mixed with blood. I wanted to help, but there was not much I could do.

So, I quietly sat on the other cot. The cell was minute, her bed so close to mine that it was impossible not to notice that she had not one vein left in her body not covered with scar tissue; a needle-poking disfigurement her addiction had caused.

It was a tragedy, and I couldn't but realize for the hundredth time that had my affair not failed, the cocaine I had brought to France necessarily would have had to circulate. Consequently, it could easily have been a part in the breakdown, if not of this particular person, perhaps of others. As a last stroke of punishment, France was giving me this daunting sight as a reminder of my transgression. By now my guilt was so deeply embedded that it was impossible to forget or forgive myself!

My confinement in Paris ended three days later. Friday May 7th, early in the morning I joined my son. Escorted by a platoon of police officers', sirens and all, John Paul and I were driven to the International Airport. Where once more we were tested to the limit. As we marched, myself cuffed to the hand of one of the escorts, John Paul handcuffed and shackled unable to be too expeditious in his walk, received only contemptuous looks from people around us.

Undeniably we were a sad sight, but the travelers' stares didn't affect us as much this time. These people didn't have a clue to all that took place in our lives, didn't realize that a tragedy such as ours could strike anyone. Humiliating still! Luckily the walk was not long. It ended in the seclusion of a private area, where Mrs. Campbell, the Canadian Consul, plus the two Canadian Mountain police officers in charge of our transfer to Canada, dressed in civilian clothes greeted us.

One of the French gendarmes handed over to the Canadian officers two large manila envelops, our documentation, files, and passports enclosed. At this point the Canadian corresponding officer firmly asked, "Will you release the handcuffs and shackles from these people now." but the French officers argued, "No, the prisoners are still in French territory. We are still in charge."

Their attitude didn't surprise us. John Paul and I knew well how vicious the French police could be and apparently even now were going to impose their rules until the very end. Except that they were in for a surprise! Just as we were, not allowing any leeway, the Mounty sternly told them. "You have released all their documentation into our hands, you no longer have any jurisdiction over them."

Reluctantly the French officers freed John Paul from the manacles and the shackles on his feet, and removed my handcuffs. It was the last we were going to hear of them! The Canadian Consul, a silent observer until then, bade us farewell wishing us the best of luck in our journey to Canada.

May 7, 1988

We boarded a 747 Jumbo Jet on a flight to Montreal. I sat next to John Paul, in the appointed seats at the tail end of the plane. The officers escorting us sat on the other side of the aisle. Nothing about them or our appearance revealed the situation.

Relief? Certainly and grateful too, but there was no way to escape the truth. We were going to Canada as convicts, carrying the heavy sentences handed to us in France. The Consul had given us an idea of what to expect in Canada. It was encouraging, except that the mark that labeled me as a criminal, invisible as it was, had left me scarred. As the plane took altitude, I closed my eyes and tried to forget wishing the flight would never end.

Some hours later the aircraft landed in Montreal and my fantasy ended. Advised beforehand by the R.C.M.P that "Everyone should disembark before we do," John Paul and I remained seated while the rest of the passengers descended. In the interval, my heart went into the erratic mode that had now become so common in me when I was not sure what to expect. Would handcuffs and shackles, sirens and flashing lights from Canadian police cars escorting us, be back on the scene?

No, none of the above; once we retrieved our luggage and reached the airport's exit terminal, only a civilian car waited for us. One of the officers broke the silence saying, "Mrs. Arthur, we'll stop first in Kingston, Ontario where the Federal Penitentiary for Woman is located. You will stay there." He then continued, this time directing his words to John Paul. "Our mission ends dropping you, in Mill-haven, the prison for men located also in Kingston. You both will be detained in those precincts, until your transfer to British Columbia is arranged."

The words were contrary to my understanding, so disappointed I spoke, "I thought everything was set for us to go all the way to Vancouver, in British Columbia." Apparently my belief had been erroneous, so not waiting for a response I asked. "Do you know when that transfer will take place?"

"No, sorry we don't."

Something unexpected had leaped in the picture and afraid of the unknown, I continued inquiring, "Will my son and I be transferred together? While we wait in those institutions, would we be able to see each other?"

Both officers shook their heads negatively, yet one of them suggested, "You need to ask those questions to the officials at the Women's Penitentiary and your son in Mill-haven. They should be able to inform you"

The drive from Montreal to Ontario took about four hours, in my view it ended too soon. The time spent next to John Paul during the transfers spoiled me; it was such a treat after the many months of being close, yet separated. At the gates of the Kingston Penitentiary, and before I descended from the car, once more I said good-by to my son hoping to see him soon, in the last stretch of our transfer

It was a Friday late in the afternoon when I was admitted in Kingston and I confronted a strange similarity to what I experienced at *Des Baumettes*; registration officials didn't work weekends. Segregation was the norm for new arrivals. Somewhat of a shocker, the inmates in the neighboring cells didn't cease to scream and bang the bars all through the night, growing louder by the minute.

However here I didn't feel threatened. I had the cell all to myself, yet for the forty-eight hours I remained in this section it was absolute madness. The outdoor break helped, even if it was just for one hour and just once a day. Still when Monday came around, I was only too happy to be placed with the rest of the population.

My introduction to the Canadian Prison for Women was intense, in more ways than I expected. Once registration was fulfilled I was directed to a cell. In the walk, I found sparkling bright hallways with shiny polished floors. Coming from Des *Baumettes* in Marseilles, it appeared that I was actually walking in a Five Star Hotel corridor!

Again I had a cell all to myself, twice as large as the ones in France. I had a bed, an enclosed bathroom with a toilet bowl and a sink; the floor and walls covered with white tiles, and I had no shower restrictions! I was still an inmate, but I felt like an incarcerated queen! Ha-ha! I had to laugh about the radical differences.

My cell as well as the others faced lengthy hallways, with the same amount of cubicle across the hall. At the front, each had iron bars from ceiling to floor, mounted on wheels. These sliding barred doors remained open during the day, giving inmates freedom of movement. At night the wheels rolled and the openings were electronically locked and the head count began. The heavy curtains at the side, were drawn shut if the occupants so desire, for bedtime privacy.

In Kingston I didn't need to recur to my fantasy to make the meals appetizing. First because it was a buffet-style cafeteria, where at breakfasts one could have a choice in the way the eggs were presented, hard boiled, fried or scrambled and sometimes omelets. Also cereals, pancakes, bacon or sausage, juices, fresh fruit, milk, coffee, tea, toast, buns and hash browns, with no limit to the servings we could have.

The choice at lunch was ample as well; salads, soups, sandwiches, juice, milk, coffee, tea and a variety of fresh fruits and deserts.

Supper! Compared to *Les Baumettes* the selection could not be more outstanding, some days roast beef, others chicken, pork chops, or fish, even stew; the serving always went with peas or corn, mashed potatoes or French fries, salads and appetizing deserts. Never a *cucaracha* or hairs, neither other uninvited guests were found. Surely for the first few days, my mouth must have dropped open in disbelief and I was in for more surprises.

Phone booth facilities! Convicted felons could use them, they only had to insert a coin and the call went through to family members, even friends. This was unheard of over in France! More implausible yet was when summoned to the Chaplain's office; he had a call waiting for me from my husband and son Patrick. It was a long distance call, the reason it required his intervention.

Likely my reaction amazed him, since all I did was cry and sob for a few minutes, before I could even say a word. Of course the chaplain didn't know that after thirty-four months, this was the first time I was hearing their voices. Once I calmed down, in between sobs I managed to hear my husband say, "I love you dear. I have already talked with John Paul and he is doing fine." John aware of the phone call privileges, made the necessary arrangements for his calls to come at a set time, every second day through the Chaplain's office.

Often I pinched myself to make sure I was not dreaming. In Kingston vs. France, inmates had a chance to take specialized courses as part of the rehabilitation programs, while professional counseling took care of psychological issues. Not to mention, the courtyard covered with green grassy areas, plus tennis, basket and volleyball courts; coming from Nice and Marseilles, how could I not think Kingston was a five-start hotel?

Yet, in the next weeks I also found negative aspects. Personally, I observed a cold aloofness and lack of compassion from guards as well as inmates; this was entirely different from what I found from the people in Nice and even in Marseilles.

I was still trying to adapt myself to my new circumstances, and hoping J.P would be benefiting from something similar, and I was notified that our transfer to B.C. had been arranged.

A Learjet! As we boarded the small jet, John Paul and I looked at each other in disbelief; our flight to Vancouver seemingly was taking place in style.

The three weeks spent confined in separate prisons were behind us now. John Paul again sat next to me and while the extent of the trip, five or six hours, I intended to shut my eyes to everything and perhaps even dream a little. Yet, how could I ignore the shackles I saw on his ankles as he difficultly shuffled his way to the plane? Or not to pay attention to the two Royal Canadian Police officers escorting us that sat in the back seats? Could I really forget the past and start living again?

The answer came soon enough, and it wasn't what I expected. As the aircraft took altitude John Paul began to talk, "Mom, I wish I didn't have to load you-up with more junk, but it's important you know what happened in Mill-heaven." Brought back to the old rough earth by my son's words, I attentively listened as in almost a whisper he reminisced the ordeal.

His expression had hardened; his beautiful olive green eyes were now petroleum green, a change that normally happened when he was either angered or sad. I didn't dare interrupt; I knew my son was about to tell me something yet very vile.

"I had been confined in segregation from day one. Let out for fresh air one hour per day, but what really got me livid was the way my situation was handled. All my meals were brought to the cell handed over by someone wearing latex gloves and through a small sliding window on the door, like you would feed a caged animal. You'll never imagined how degraded I felt. It was actually hateful. What kept me going was to know that our transfer to British Columbia was in the works. I certainly hope I don't have to go through the same at Kent."

My son's words hurt as if someone had sliced my heart with vengeance. Such callous behavior troubled me. Once more my son was the expiratory lamb. It appeared that we had come out from one horror story into another of another kind.

As if trying to ease the duress of the last events he experienced, gently and with a smile John Paul spoke again, "Not all was bad, Mom. I was seen by the prison's physician twice; who after evaluating the tests run on me and comparing with the files brought from France said, "You are fine, John Paul." At that point I could not but ask him, "Why then am I treated in this manner? In short I explained how differently my situation was handled in France."

He simple told me, "I will tell you this much John Paul, in Canada the general public doesn't know much about the HIV virus, or AIDS. Some don't take it kindly; they hold the idea that anyone can be contaminated by a simple touch. I suggest you don't mention anything about it when you get to the next place. The least guards an inmates know about your condition, the less chance you'll have to be treated in the same manner, elsewhere. I believe you are going to Kent, right? There, neither you nor your mother should volunteer information about your health. Higher authorities have your file; they'll examine it and make an intelligent decision based on the information provided."

"Do you understand why I'm bringing all this up, Mom? We have to be cautious, it's best if we don't mention anything about my ailment, or write about it in future letters, okay?" I certainly acceded. It appeared that in Canada being HIV positive had deeper ramifications. Necessarily we had to be more vigilant in the text of our letters! The rest of the flight proceeded calmly and uncomplicated.

Actually the Mounties treated us with civility, unlike France under similar circumstances; but now no matter how positively I wanted to think, all was still too conflictive. For the moment the only strong and solid matter was our repatriation and relocation, thanks to my husband's love and tenacity.

Hard to believe that not too long ago, my life had been so different; when indictments, sentences and prisons were not in the picture. A time abundant with love, respect and admiration; an epoch where I hardly had any worries and when we were a happy family, now just a mirage from the past!

Yet I knew that all the misery we went through, had not broken our core, it had forged us stronger instead; ready to contend with whatever the future wanted to bring us. As if to reinforce my thoughts, the incredible beauty of British Columbia embraced us now, there was something exhilarating in the air. While the drive to my new destination in a Sheriff's vehicle, John Paul and I saw the multicolored and exuberant vegetation, flowers everywhere; maple trees and other green forestry in the background as if greeting us, giving us a new hope.

Informed beforehand, John Paul and I knew our new destinations; John Paul was going to Kent a Federal maximum-security penitentiary about one hour from Mission, where John and Patrick lived now. As we agreed in the plane, J. P. and I would keep quiet about his ailment and pray for the best, and added that in a short time he was to be released on Full Parole and join his father and brother, I had no great trepidations about his well being. So without tears this time, I bade my son farewell.

Since British Columbia lacked Federal penitentiaries for women, after intensive paper work that started at the Canadian Embassy in France, and continued in Kingston, I was accepted to serve whatever part of my sentence was left at Lake-view a Provincial Correctional Institution for women, known better by the name of Okala in Burnaby (now no longer in existence).

Otherwise my destination would have been somewhere in Alberta, where the only Federal Prison for women closer to home was located. At this point I didn't comprehend the differences between the two systems Provincial and Federal, it would be a while before I did. Yet thanks to the diligence and help of so many superb Canadian persons in office, I was now in B. C. about one hour away from our home in Mission.

Seemingly Okala was just a transition place before I relocated once more. Unknown exactly when this would happened, nothing was programmed for exterior visits, therefore I would have to wait a bit longer before I saw my husband and younger son again. In the mean time two unexpected but constructive events lighten up the wait. A new Guardian Angel came knocking on my door, Father McDonald, the Catholic chaplain, who later on would prove to be of great consequence on the road to freedom.

The other one had to do with work, I'm not too sure how or why, but a lot of laundering was performed in Okala. So every morning after breakfast I unloaded the dryers and neatly folded all the stuff out of them, the majority was bedding. Shown by other inmates the how, I became an expert in folding fitted sheets. However my training was soon interrupted.

My international transfer ended at Twin Maples, a minimum-security complex that turned out to be another unusual correctional institution. My surprise was greater yet than what I experienced in Kingston; a farm at one time, the establishment later had been transformed into a detention center, added portable units supplemented the room space. Situated at only 30 minutes from Mission, where John had purchased a house and soon to be my home too.

Here I shared a bedroom with other three detainees, we all had comfortable beds nicely covered with colorful bedspreads, a small dresser for each and there was and adjacent bathroom for our use. The large farmhouse must have had at least ten bedrooms a spacious kitchen and just as large dining area.

Two of the portable units served as recreation centers, one with some table games, and the other with a big television set and a VCR, both regularly full after dinner. One more unit was set as a schoolroom with eight or ten computers; a teacher came twice a week, to teach us the basics plus some math.

All 40 detainees worked, it was mandatory. The reason was to teach us a pattern to be followed once we were released to the life outside. The pay was four dollars and fifty cents per day, remuneration mainly for canteen expenditures, such as special treats, cosmetics, cigarettes and other superfluous things not provided by the institution, but certainly not beer!

The times we were not working or in class, as well as in the evenings, inmates had freedom of mobility within the farm. A little ways from the main area, a craft shop was available, where a coach guided us to work with clay, mold and fired beautiful ceramic artifacts. Where later and after some failures, I managed to make a mug for my husband that once cocked was white with John's name in black, inscribed in the object; the artwork was therapeutically great.

The farm itself had a barn, a tractor, a few cows, five or six horses, the same amount of pigs, and some chickens and ducks. Inmates who wanted to work with the livestock looked after the animals and some worked in the small greenhouse. Not me, it was not my calling.

Four others and myself worked in the kitchen, under the instruction and supervision of a hired professional cook. I chose this job because the workload was within a specific period of time. I got up at 5 am but it gave me enough free time in the morning after breakfast, and in the afternoon before supper to brainstorm a bit in the computer world and art.

It was here that without any red tape, I saw my husband and Patrick for the first time after almost 36 months of no physical contact. I was kissed and hugged by both, and I hugged and kissed both back, again and again, I couldn't believe the incredible reality that I was now living. I held their faces with both my hands, making sure it was not a dream. We shed tears, and laughed.

Patrick was now almost 18, and a very handsome young man. Blue eyes, about 5'10, blond wavy hair, a bit long. I supposed he went with the trend of the day and actually he looked good with the slightly long hair. I had missed so much of his growing up years; I'd left him only a child and now he was a man.

John and Patrick came every other day after 6 pm, the hour at which supper and the chores at the farm were completed. Sundays the doors opened at 2 and we spent part of the afternoon together, within the grounds of the facility. Benches and tables made it look more like a park than a Correctional Institution. The other days and times, my two loved ones went to visit J. P.

Twin Maples brought to my life something that I had almost forgot existed: unlocked doors, unlocked gates! Freedom was one step away. It was tempting, but I was able to hold back thanks to my husband and younger son, who regularly stopped by to see me, always bringing fresh news from John Paul, and where I also enjoyed Father McDonald's visits. He became my friend and spiritual guide.

As Father McDonald took a liking to me, one day he asked me, "Would you mind if I brought a couple of friends? They are involved with the justice system, one is a Judge from Australia and the other is the Regional Chaplain for the Pacific Region of the CSC. I have mentioned to them what you have told me, not in the secret of confession, but the other part of your story and conviction. My friends are very interested and would like to meet you, if that is alright with you?"

Of course I didn't mind, and I met them. In a personal note they found the sentences given to us in France extremely harsh, compared to similar cases in Australia and Canada. Later the Regional Chaplain, whose mandate was also Parole Supervision and management of the parole office, would become John Paul's Parole officer.

June 15, 1988

Dearest Mother,

We are here; we finally made it! Never felt better in my life since 1985. Upon my arrival in Kent, I was put with the rest of the inmate population. No more segregation, no more of the junk I went through in Mill-haven. I hope that in that fabulous farm, you too are finding everything better than what you anticipated.

The surroundings around this place are beautiful; mountains in the background and very peaceful. I understand the nearest town, located five minutes from Kent, has only fifteen hundred inhabitants. I have a cell all to myself. We eat in a great restaurant similar to the one you found at the Five Star Hotel. Remember you told me about it on the plane, while I only complained. Ha, ha. I can laugh about it now!

Though there is something puzzling in this place; I don't quite understand the disposition most of the inmates have, if any one of them finds you talking in a cordial manner with the guards as we used to do in France, immediately you feel a wave of hostility. Their anger is overpowering. I find it absurd; guards are only people doing their jobs. Oh well, each to their own.

Something else I found funny around here is that at mealtime, you can't sit wherever you please unless you are specifically invited. Some boys seem to hold ownership over the spaces, and if anyone accidentally or not, occupies one of those places, you risk a beating. Luckily for me, I only experienced the contrary; I am always invited to the club. Ha, ha.

Seriously now, I found out that any money sent from outside is put in a special account but we are not able to use it; kind like a savings? So right now I don't have enough, to purchase the materials I need to continue with my art. It does not mean that I don't have enough for my personal needs, because as you know we get paid four dollars and fifty cents per day, either for going to school or working. I'm going to school.

Someone told me that I could earn the extra money by selling some of the drawings I brought from France. So, when Dad comes next time I will ask him to buy them, I am sure he will be happy to do it. Then once I have the materials I need, I will prepare more pieces for the Art Exhibition the Institution lets inmates have in July.

Mom, I always wanted to ask you something but I did not know how. Now I would like to do it. Are you ready for life outside prison's walls? I understand you are afraid, afraid even of open spaces after the two and a half years of confinement. I feel a bit the same myself, but it is important we overcome these fears.

Remember that we are not losers, Mom; we are fighters. Besides we don't have anything to be ashamed of. It was all a big mistake but that is it. We have paid more than enough and God knows it. I am sure He wants us to start a new life. You *certainly must feel His protection, as I do. So, smile and do a good job in preparing the request for your parole.*

Patrick and Dad both need us strong, not a pair of weak crybabies. Remember we are on the homestretch. I am very proud of my family. The love that you, Dad and Patrick have always shown me has helped me adapt to each new situation. May God bless you all, over and over; we must praise Him and never again fear for our safety. He will look after us.

Once I am in Ferndale, the minimum-security place, I believe we will be allowed to visit each other. It seems that escort passes are authorized, so I will probably be seeing you soon.

I love you Mother, J. P.

P.S. Good news! I don't have to wait much longer here, the nineteenth is my transfer to Ferndale.

It was the last letter I would have from my J.P. Thereafter we communicated by phone. Not as often nor as long as the other inmates, who connected with their family and friends in the exterior, using the pay phones set for that purpose but not to buzz prisoners in other correctional institutions. Our situation fitted in this last phase. As a result, twice a week the officials in charge of our files placed the calls for us, and John Paul and I voiced our mutual concerns over the phone instead.

The humanity I personally experienced at the farm was somewhat similar to the warmth I received in Nice, and didn't stop there. Patrick, who just finished high school, had his graduation day June 27. Anne my case manager, supportive to the idea of the benefit I would obtain by being at the ceremony, procured and granted me an escorted day pass to attend the event; my husband was my designated escort.

Dressed appropriately for the occasion with the outfit I made at the workshop, I waited at the farm for my date, John. He picked me up about one hour ahead of the ceremony and in his car I was driven to the High School in Mission. It was my first outing almost as a free woman, and no less than to be present on a such memorable day in our younger son's life, without a sentinel on sight to ruin the moment. We looked and were just as any other couple, and very proud parents.

All was good, yet I had a let down to my dreams when on August 1988, after I applied for a conditional release before the Provincial Parole Board I was granted only a Day Parole. The four gentlemen from the board, never before had dealt with a situation like mine; their expertise lay in offenders sentenced to terms less than two years, nothing to do with lengthily ones like mine. It was here where the difference between Provincial and Federal systems lay. Had they known more about Federal offenses and the complexity of my case, I am sure they would have granted me a Full Parole.

Hurt but thankful, I complied with my Conditional Release provisos; which it stipulated that for the next thirty months, 2 ½ more years, I would reside in a half-way house for women in Vancouver under strict regulations; for one to be back at the residence always before the 20 hundred hour, the curfew time! The Elizabeth Fry Society, a Christian agency, was in charge of the house's management.

The second one stipulated that I should find work to support myself, a condition I was only too eager to abide, particularly after all the expenses incurred in France. Other than I was not ready to interact with persons in the free world, I believe it was written all over my face that I was a convict. Matters got even tougher when my criminal record had to be known by whoever employed me. Which made me question, who in the world would want to hire an ex-convict?

Even so, the staff in Twin Maples had helped me prepare a resume with details of my work experience, business management, typing and computer skills. It looked good on paper, but it didn't do much to uplift my spirit or wipe away the blemish and my embarrassment. John Paul, who sensed my inadequacy, wrote encouragement words on his last letter in an effort to help me overcome the negative; yet I still struggled with it.

In succession I was linked to another governmental agency, who connected me with a reputable accountant, owner of several small business in Vancouver. I had an interview with him. Somehow I found the courage to tell him everything. Surprisingly, I was hired.

John Paul's file on the contrary did not take long to be examined by the National Parole Board and because of his non-criminality record and medical condition, on August 16 1988 he was given a Full Parole by Exception, prior to his normal eligibility. The gentleman I met in Twin Maples, introduced by father McDonald, became John Paul's Parole officer, and J.P. reported to him once a month. My son then moved in with his father and brother.

Health wise John Paul was still holding his own, but he thought out the processional advise of a well known G.P in Vancouver. Who suggested that he should take specific supplements, which should help sustain and fortify his immune system. From then on the doctor saw John Paul regularly and to complement the agenda my son joined in a gym and began a bodybuilding program.

Not like a dream anymore, everything was coming in place. John found and excellent job in his field, sold the house in Mission and relocated my family to Abbotsford. John Paul and Patrick with the backing of their father started to build a few speck homes that once were completed, quickly sold; the strong real estate market helped. One of the houses was kept as the family's dwelling and the two boys purchased two more lots, under builder's terms and continued on the business of building.

Whereas my one and only desire was to be with my family and help, but the restrictions of my Day Parole and my work schedule obstructed the actuality of my dream. I started to work at half past twelve mid day and ended at nine pm, just one more hour before my curfew time; this together with the one hour plus drive between Abbotsford and Vancouver, held me captive.

Even so, the three men in life resourceful as ever, found a remedy. Saturday and Sundays, my husband, John Paul, and Patrick came to Vancouver to take me out. In Quesnel, John had purchased a second-hand vehicle, a station wagon big as boat and put into perfect condition by his stepdad; it was used now in our expeditions.

In that vessel we toured around Vancouver. None of us was yet familiar with the metropolis, but in no time with the help of a good road map we got to know almost every corner of the town. Nevertheless, by ten o'clock, like Cinderella before my coach turned into a pumpkin, dutifully I returned to my cage.

Some months later the Fry society fulfilling the parole's long-term plan allowed me to have overnight sleeps on Saturdays. Early in the morning on that day, either John Paul or Patrick came to pick me up and I had the joy to spend the weekends at home. At this point is when my mother and sister came for a visit.

We had a grand family reunion; we shed many tears, but they were happy ones this time, though at one point I disclosed our secret to my sister, not to Mom yet. There was no need to cause her more suffering; she had more than enough with our imprisonment. Vicky then understood the desperate steps I took, trying to save my son, and finally I got her total forgiveness. Mother stayed permanently; my husband's promise that we would look after her turned into a fact, and part of my dream became a reality. It did not matter that much if the rest of the week, I still lived at the Halfway House. Vicky after a month with us flew back to her family.

One Sunday in the later part of September, when I still visited my family only on the weekends, love came knocking on our door. I knew Patrick had a steady relationship with a girl and this particular day, our younger son brought the young lady to meet us. She was about his own age, and very attractive; I sensed she was also beautiful inside. I liked her, we all did. It was easy to be fond of her. Pam then began to take part in our outings, but we didn't share all our secrets with her not just yet.

While John Paul who felt great, health wise, decided to pursue other interests. With the tourism background he picked up from Judith in France, plus his domain in French, he was offered an excellent job as a Tourist Consultant. The work involved traveling to Montreal and Ontario, to bring and guide tourists from the old continent to Alberta and British Columbia.

Once he obtained the necessary permission for this travels from his parole officer, John Paul worked productively in the tourist industry, but this new career prompted him to move to Vancouver. So we saw him frequently, but not as often as before.

Patrick, who by then had created his own construction company, kept building houses quite successfully and still does. His relationship with Pam continued with goals to get married in a near future.

On Jan 2nd, 1990, thanks to a review of the remission in the sentencing time given by France, I was granted Full Parole. At last I was able to jump on board and find work closer to home. Except that having been conditioned for far too long by Penitentiaries, Correctional Systems, halfway houses, etc., it still troubled me to freely talk to people or make friends. What if they found I had criminal past and rejected me?

In my view friendships were built on love and trust. I was eager to give my love, but my criminal record and my son's illness inhibited me to disclose my secrets; my trust at this point was virtually zero. Besides I also felt that keeping silent about my past was almost the same as lying, so I chose to remain in my own protective cocoon around my family, always with a watchful eye on John Paul's health..

Yet I knew a job to help in our finances was a must for me, so after taking an upgrading course in nursing I found work. I became a Home Support Worker taking care of the elderly and disabled people in their homes. From the start, I told the agency's manager about my criminal record. Kate, likewise my previous boss, gave me the chance to prove my trustworthiness. I began September 1990.

Supposedly it takes twenty-one days to break an old habit, and about the same to change into a new good one. I am sure it took a lot longer for me to readapt to a life of almost total freedom; I still had to report once a month to my parole officer.

In the mist of these internal battles with myself, one day when John Paul came to visit us, I sensed something troubling my oldest son but ignorant of the ramifications my question would bring, I asked him, "Is there anything wrong John Paul? You seem sad."

"Mom it's very hard for me to bring up this subject, but I can't keep hiding it or deny it any more. Besides I know you will find out sooner or later; so I think it is best if you learned directly from me. You might have even guessed it already; I'm gay, Mom!"

John Paul spoke those words fast and furiously, as if he didn't say his piece now, he would never say it. While I just stared at him, my son kept talking, "I can't help it Mom. The Lord knows I tried! But, I have to start living my life the way it is, and stop lying to myself as well as to you all. I have a partner now. His name is Andrew. He knows I'm HIV positive, he is too." Cold perspiration ran through my body as I assimilated my son's words, unable to say anything, the same as a few years a go.

Did I really sense it? Had this knowledge been buried deep down in my subconscious and I ignored it. Had I been in denial all these years? It was possible. At the time when John Paul told me that he had contracted the malady through having sex with prostitutes, candidly I wanted to believe his story. Except that I

384 | MYRIAM ARTHUR

now knew I accepted my own interpretation of the story because I really didn't want to know the truth, then all the rest piled on us.

My first reaction after the shock was to open my arms and embraced him. He was my son and I loved him dearly, no matter what and I knew my love would be forever. Besides, who was I to judge anyway?

I was speechless, other than to say, "I love you honey; no matter what I will always love you John Paul." Rapidly I excused myself, saying, "I must run to the bank now, I have business to attend to." Instead I went to church. I drove to Saint Ann's Catholic Church in tears and fear. It was the parish I now attended, although I didn't yet have a spiritual guide.

My years in France had brought me back to the Lord, but I knew that some Christian churches had controversial opinions about homosexuality. What if my Church considered sinful that I still loved my son, even after he told me that he was a homosexual? Yet, at the same time I believed it would be impossible for a true Church in Christ, to think that way.

Was not God himself, love? Had not the Lamb of God been sacrificed for prodigal sons and daughters as well as righteous ones? Fair questions and answers, but it was important for me that I learn the point of view of the Catholic Church on this particular subject.

My tears kept pouring down while I drove, while I also prayed. Not really knowing what I was praying for, but I soon realized I was asking God, more than anything for His guidance on the attitude my family and I should adopt towards John Paul.

I rang the bell at Saint Ann's. A few seconds later a short man, wearing a priest's white collar opened the door and with a warm smile on his face and a strong Spanish accent said, "I am Father Santiago Suarez, the new helping priest, what can I do for you?" I firmly believe God placed Father Santiago at Saint Ann's parish, at this particular moment in my life to be my guide, to direct my walk in the most difficult of trials I still had ahead of me.

After Father Santiago heard me, he said, "There is no conflict with the love you have for your son and the Church. God loves every one of us, with our faults and inadequacies. The Church as his spouse supports Christ's teachings; love and forgiveness equally for everyone, prodigal sons or daughters included."

"You can be at peace with yourself, Myriam, because I'm sure God will never be opposed to the most beautiful sentiment such as the love a mother and father have for their child. Doesn't He have just that for all of us? I suggest you let John Paul know you love him. He needs to hear it, now more than ever before." The priest's words gave the peace I needed.

This time I shared what I learned about our son with John, and my husband embracing me simply said, "I had guessed it for a long time honey, but I didn't feel comfortable bringing the subject up with you." We didn't discuss the issued any further, but I knew John loved John Paul just the same; our son's admission, had not affected my husband's feelings either. We never stopped showing our affection and accepted his friend Andrew into our home.

Life continued on and in the hands of the excellent doctor and a cocktail of medications that he had added to his daily intake, John Paul kept well.

Since mother was staying in Canada permanently, it was necessary to put a closure to her affairs in Bolivia. She still had her condo and the place was totally unnecessary, it had to be sold. A real state agency could easily have handled the sale, however when mother sold the big house, most all her belongings moved with her, some were put in storage; all will need to be sorted out.

Therefore a trip to Bolivia was essential, but my mother at her age couldn't travel alone, or rummage through the personal belongings of a lifetime by herself. As much as I hated the idea, it was imperative I went along with her and in the way pick up my sister from Lima; we both needed to be involved. Yet the conditions of my Parole didn't allow me to leave the country. The Regional Chaplain that I met at the Maple farm who by now knew my entire family well, put a good word in favor and my own

Parole officer accepted my request and granted permission to travel back to my country.

After almost seven years of absence, the second week of November 1992 I arrived in Cochabamba, together with my mother and sister; they both were conscious of my dismay to face everyone in my city. The whole town, I mean the persons who knew me, all were aware of what took place in France. Some wrote to me, others gave the support to my mother, but this would be the first time I would be facing them and I was embarrassed to say the least.

My cousin Raul, who knew of our arrival, was the first to come with his wife to wish us well. Through him, other cousins and friends that learned we were in town also came and we were invited to family gatherings or tea reunions with other friends. No one ever asked anything about France, or made malicious comments about my incarceration. Instead all opened their arms in profound friendship.

Not Mauricio, our old friend and partner; I supposed still scalded by the whole thing didn't make an appearance. My prolonged silence after his first letters, and perhaps by whatever situation the dissolution of the partnership created, John never gave me any details, remained out of sight!

Curious, but more than anything remorseful, after all my action had harmed him and the damage had extended to the company too, I tried to reach out and I called him.

Ring Ring the phone buzzed and Mauricio answered. "Hello?" he said and when I identified myself, harshly Mauricio reproached me, "So finally you decide to show up." As if it was up to me to be accessible all this time. It was not the response or the tone in which he said those words that I had expected. Immediately my good intentions disappeared and my pride, the old stuff which I thought I lost it while imprisoned, kicked in again and not thinking twice on the spot, I hung up the receiver. I never heard from him, nor Mauricio would hear from me again; our friendship had died and was now buried.

The condo sold quickly and very swiftly we went through everything to decide what we wanted to keep for safekeeping; we sold or gave away the rest. Generous as ever Mom again gave my sister and I the sum of $30,000 each and kept a smaller amount for herself. These moneys were respectively wired to banks in Canada and Peru.

Mother and I, after a short stay at my sister's place, returned to Canada only to learn that John Paul had been admitted to St. Paul's hospital with pneumonia. His doctor, who now had specialized in HIV matters, treated him with a powerful dose of antibiotics in order to control the infection.

John Paul recovered and was well for his brother's wedding with Pamela. It took place May 29 1993; John Paul was the best man. After the wedding Pam's parents offered a reception, which we all enjoyed.

John Paul had rented a condo by the beach in Vancouver, and some Sundays all of us visited him, and spent the day swimming in the cool waters of English Bay. He continued to work, however his health began to decline. By November of the same year, the month of his birthday, he was down with pneumonia once again, and under the antibiotic treatment to some extent John Paul improved. Enough to be able to join us with Andrew, December 24th, for the family gathering I traditionally held to celebrate the Nativity of our Lord Jesus.

First we attended mass at St. Ann, and once back at home we all sat down to eat the meal I had prepared. We were eight at the table, Mom, John and I, John Paul and Andrew, Patrick and Pamela and our guest of honor Father Santiago. Later with great camaraderie we opened the presents.

Right after New Year's Day, John Paul became seriously ill, with major complications in his digestive system was again admitted into the Vancouver hospital. His depleted immune system did not respond to the medication and the disease kept on its destructive course. January came and went, then February, and there were no signs of improvement, on the contrary dehydration had set in, and his lungs were also compromised; the I.V. treatment that he had on going 24/7 was not helping.

A recovery could only come through a miracle; I kept on praying for one to happen. Father Thomas, the Catholic Chaplain at St. Paul, who constantly sat by J. P.'s bedside, tendered not only for my son's spiritual needs but also was a great humane contact for him and a veiled blessing for me. Father Thomas and father Santiago watched over all of us through out these hours of need.

Monday through Friday, after work and once we finished the evening meal, I set off to see my son, often bringing him home-made soup, some of John Paul's favorites. He always enjoyed the soup and now it was the only thing he was able to swallow without throwing up. Usually John and my mother came along, but the one-hour plus drive from Abbotsford into Vancouver and the hour back to our town was becoming a bit hard on my Mom.

My husband, who didn't need to return to his work in Mexico just yet, unselfishly chose to stay with her at home. He knew of the strong fixation I had to check on my son daily, no matter what. John's support was extraordinary, but I already knew how great of a man he was, even more now that I saw him put his own feelings and needs aside, so that my most fervent desire to be with John Paul was fulfilled.

It would have been easy for me to request a leave of absence from work. Except that we now had an added mortgage to our household expenses and my income even if not vital, was necessary to fill in the gap. Later in March, John Paul's condition dramatically deteriorated and I turned my evening visits into overnight stays; if the prayer for miracle didn't come soon, I did not know for how much longer our son would be with us.

The nurses aware of my unbreakable need kindly set a recliner chair next to John Paul's bed for my comfort and just before the sun was up, after I gently kissed my son's forehead, I quietly left. The 75 km drive that early in the morning, was no problem, there was hardly any traffic and within one hour I was home.

The minute I arrived, I checked on my mother, who was just getting up. I gave a huge kiss to my husband, thanked him for all he was doing to help me out, and presented him a detailed account on John Paul's night. I then had a shower, put on a clean set of clothes, made breakfast and once I swallowed the last bite, off I went to work and came back for lunch. It was my daily routine. I didn't think anything of it; I was just doing what needed to be done.

One morning after John Paul had been restless all through the night and therefore me too, driving in the fast lane on the Trans-Canada Highway heading for home as usual, my eyelids became very heavy. I opened the window to have some fresh air on my face and even slapped my cheeks to keep me alert. Yet it was getting harder and harder to keep my eye lids open; fortunately in only two more exists, I would be home, I thought.

Suddenly I found myself driving in the meridian, apparently overcome by the heaviness of my eyelids, within seconds I went down in the embankment onto the terrain that divided the East/ West Highway. However once I realized what was happening, I was able to control the steering wheel and maneuver the vehicle onto flat land; my heart beating just as fast as the Buick.

Probably in shock, I forgot to pull my foot off the gas pedal or who knows; but the car had not rolled over and for seconds I thought I had conquered the problem. I only had to step on the brake pedal and stop the vehicle, but the plan didn't work. The Buick hit, head-on, a draining ditch that ran transversally. I must have fainted with the impact and as I regained consciousness, I heard someone saying, "Don't move, the ambulance will be here in a minute."

Soon the ambulance attendants carefully pulled me out of the car; which later I learned was a total wreck. It appears that with the collision the air bag exploded, pushing my body against the seat, protecting me from being propelled out through the front window. Once out of the wreck, and placed on a stretcher I was taken to the hospital with sirens and all! At my request one of the attendees called my husband and informed him of the accident.

While examined and X-rayed at the E.R. every piece of my body ached, but I found that my injuries were not as bad as what it could have been. The doctor in turn told me, "You have three compressed lumbar vertebrae, the L3-L4 and L5. You need to be immobile for a few days and you will be all right; I'll have you transferred as an inpatient to the main wing." John who had just arrived heard the diagnosis and agreed with the doctor.

Not me; I had other plans. I was not going to be hospitalized while my son might be on his deathbed in a Vancouver hospital; it was not going to happen. At once and almost in a whisper I told my husband, "You are going to get me out of here now. I am not staying!" Then addressing the doctor I said, "I really don't need to stay. I promise to rest and be immobile at home; it will be better for me. I have an elderly mother that I look after and she needs me around her, otherwise it will too stressful for both of us."

The physician could not detain me, as it would be going against my wishes. As a result he had no other alternative than to prescribe some painkillers and release me. John unaware yet of what I had in mind and convinced that I was going to do just as what I had told the doctor, helped me get dressed. However as I was getting down from the bed, I felt an agonizing pain in my lower back. It almost made me black out, but I was not going to let that stop me. John stood next to me, so I grabbed his arm and told him, "Honey support me please. I need your help to walk."

Once out, I explained what I had in mind. "John, you know how ill our son is. I can't stay in Abbotsford while he might be dying; I need to be next to him. So this is what we will do. Let's pick up Mom and few clothes for myself and then you are going to drive me to Vancouver. You saw the recliner chair the nurses have put next to John Paul's bed for me. I will rest and be immobile there, promise. I will be fine dear, you will see." John tried to dissuade me, but with no luck. So I moved into the Vancouver hospital March 15th.

My sister, aware of the situation, came to help with Mom and to give us all moral support. My decision was more satisfying, now I didn't need to leave my son's side for anything, except to go to the bathroom or have a quick shower. My back hurt but it didn't matter. John, my mother, and sister came every day, as well as Patrick and Pam.

Every one of us was aware that the end was near, John Paul was in agony. My prayers for his recovery became now prayers for the Lord to take my son home with Him; father Thomas had already administered the last rites. I couldn't see John Paul suffer any more. I had to let him go!

John Paul died April 11, 1994 at Saint Paul's Hospital, surrounded by the love of his entire family; my Mom, John, my sister, Patrick and Pamela, Andrew and myself.

Epilogue

IT WAS AN IRREPARABLE LOSS FOR ALL, AND NONE MORE SO THAN for me. Do I have any regrets? No I don't, I had done my best, even if my best sometimes was wrong. I had experienced incredible moments of closeness with John Paul and with my family. Right or wrong it was all done out of love. I do miss my son John Paul. I know he has forgiven me for the afflictions he experienced because of my wrong. I am also aware that my entire family has forgiven me too for the pain and anxiety my wrong caused. Most importantly, I also know the Lord has forgiven me.

Even Canada, my adopted country forgave me. May 7, 2003 the National Parole Board awarded me a Pardon on my criminal record and after making the proper inquires, and were satisfied that I had remained free of any convictions since the completion of my sentence and that I was of good conduct, included the five years of the waiting period on indictable offenses.

Yet to entirely close the book on this episode of our lives, it would necessary that I learn to forgive the blindness and injustice of the French justice system, which I believe will never happen.

However, poetic justice was served. Four years later, after our transferred to Canada I came to learn that the District Attorney, Monsieur Clavier had been murdered and I then remembered

John Paul's prophetic words when we were still undergoing his interrogation game:

"The man is insane. One day he will render account for all the cruelty he is leaving behind! Be sure of that Mom!"

The End

CPSIA information can be obtained at www.ICGtesting.com
Printed in the USA
LVOW08s0803061113

360122LV00001B/11/P